Rapid Weight Loss Hypnosis

The Most Complete Guide for Women on How to Lose Weight Effortlessly and Naturally through Proven Self-Hypnosis Techniques, Affirmations and Guided Meditations

2 Manuscripts in 1 Book

Elizabeth Collins

Rapid Weight Loss Hypnosis for Women

Table of Contents

Introduction

Hypnosis is rewiring your brain to add or to change your daily routine starting from your basic instincts. This happens due to the fact that while you are in a hypnotic state you are more susceptible to suggestions by the person who put you in this state. In the case of self-hypnosis, the person who made you enter the trance of hypnotism is yourself. Thus, the only person who can give you suggestions that can change your attitude in this method is you and you alone.

Again, you must forget the misconception that hypnosis is like sleeping because if it is then it would be impossible to give autosuggestions to yourself. Try to think about it like being in a very vivid daydream where you are capable of controlling every aspect of the situation you are in. This gives you the ability to change anything that may bother and hinder you to achieve the best possible result. If you are able to pull it off properly, then the possibility of improving yourself after a constant practice of the method will just be a few steps away.

Career

People say that motivation is the key to improve in your career. But no matter how you love your career, you must admit that there are aspects in your work that you really do not like doing. Even if it is a fact that you are good in the other tasks, there is that one duty that you dread. And every time you encounter this specific chore you seem to be slowed down and thus lessening your productivity at work. This is where self-hypnosis comes into play.

The first thing you need to do is find that task you do not like. In some cases there might be multiple of them depending on your personality and how you feel about your job. Now, try to look at why you do not like that task and do simple research on how to make the job a lot simpler. You can then start conditioning yourself to use the simple method every time you do the job.

After you are able to condition your state of mind to do the task, each time you encounter it will become the trigger for your trance and thus giving you the ability to perform it better. You will not be able to tell the difference since you will not mind it at all. Your coworkers and superiors though will definitely notice the change in your work style and in your productivity.

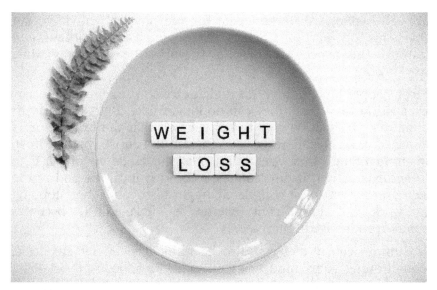

Family

It is easy to improve in a career. But to improve your relationship with your family can be a little tricky. Yet, self-hypnosis can still reprogram you to interact with your family members better by modifying how you react to the way they act. You will have the ability to adjust your way of thinking depending on the situation. This then allows you to respond in the most positive way possible, no matter how dreadful the scenario may be.

If you are in a fight with your husband/wife, for example, the normal reaction is to flare up and face fire with fire. The problem with this approach is it usually engulfs the entire relationship which might eventually lead up to separation. Being in a hypnotic state in this instance can help you think clearly and change the impulse of saying the words without thinking through. Anger will still be there, of course, that is the healthy way. But anger now under self-hypnosis can be channeled and stop being a raging inferno, you can turn it into a steady bonfire that can help you and your partner find common ground for whatever issue you are facing. The same applies in dealing with a sibling or children. If you are able to condition your mind to think more rationally or to get into the perspective of others, then you can have better family/friends' relationships.

Health and Physical Activities

Losing weight can be the most common reason why people will

use self-hypnosis in terms of health and physical activities. But this is just one part of it. Self-hypnosis can give you a lot more to improve this aspect of your life. It works the same way while working out.

Most people tend to give up their exercise program due to the exhaustion they think they can no longer take. But through self-hypnosis, you will be able to tell yourself that the exhaustion is lessened and thus allowing you to finish the entire routine. Keep in mind though that your mind must never be conditioned to forget exhaustion, it must only not mind it until the end of the exercise. Forgetting it completely might lead you to not stopping to work out until your energy is depleted. It becomes counterproductive in this case.

Having a healthy diet can also be influenced by self-hypnosis. Conditioning your mind to avoid unhealthy food can be done. Thus, hypnosis will be triggered each you are tempted to eat a meal you are conditioned to consider as unhealthy. Your eating habit then can change to benefit you to improve your overall health.

Mental, Emotional and Spiritual Needs

Since self-hypnosis deals directly in how you think, it is then no secret that it can greatly improve your mental, emotional and spiritual needs. A clear mind can give your brain the ability to have more rational thoughts. Rationality then leads to better decision making and easy absorption and retention of information you might need to improve your mental capacity. You must set your expectations, though; this does not work like magic that can turn you into a genius. The process takes time depending on how far you want to go, how much you want to achieve. Thus, the effects will only be limited by how much you are able to condition your mind.

In terms of emotional needs, self-hypnosis cannot make you feel differently in certain situations. But it can condition you to take in each scenario a little lighter and make you deal with them better. Others think that getting rid of emotion can be the best course of action if you are truly able to rewire your brain. But they seem to forget that even though rational thinking is often influenced negatively by emotion, it is still necessary for you to decide on things basing on the common ethics and aesthetics of the real world. Self-hypnosis then can channel your emotion to work in a more positive way in terms of decision making and dealing with emotional hurdles and problems.

Spiritual need on the other hand is far easier to influence when it comes to doing self-hypnosis. As a matter of fact, most people with spiritual beliefs are able to do self-hypnosis each time they practice what they believe in. A deep prayer, for instance, is a way to self-hypnotize yourself to enter the trance to feel closer to a Divine existence. Chanting and meditation done by other religions also leads and have the same goal. Even the songs during a mass or praise and worship triggers self-hypnosis depending if the person allows them to do so.

Still, the improvements can only be achieved if you condition yourself that you are ready to accept them. The willingness to put an effort must also be there. An effortless hypnosis will only create the illusion that you are improving and thus will not give you the satisfaction of achieving your goal in reality.

How hypnosis can help resolve childhood issues

Another issue that hypnosis can help you with are problems from our past. If you have had traumatic situations from your childhood days, then you may have issues in all areas of your adult life. Unresolved issues from your past can lead to anxiety and depression in your later years. Childhood trauma is dangerous because it can alter many things in the brain both psychologically and chemically.

The most vital thing to remember about trauma from your childhood is that given a harmless and caring environment in which the child's vital needs for physical safety, importance, emotional security and attention are met, the damage that trauma and abuse cause can be eased and relieved. Safe and dependable relationships are also a dynamic component in healing the effects of childhood trauma in adulthood and make an atmosphere in which the brain can safely start the process of recovery.

Pure Hypnoanalysis is the lone most effective method of treatment available in the world today, for the resolution of phobias, anxiety, depression, fears, psychological and emotional problems/symptoms and eating disorders. It is a highly advanced form of hypnoanalysis (referred to as analytical hypnotherapy or hypno-analysis). Hypnoanalysis, in its numerous forms, is practiced all over the world; this method of hypnotherapy can completely resolve the foundation of anxieties in the unconscious mind, leaving the individual free of their symptoms for life.

There is a deeper realism active at all times around us and inside us. This reality commands that we must come to this world to find happiness, and every so often that our inner child stands in our way. This is by no means intentional; however, it desires to reconcile wounds from the past or address damaging philosophies which were troubling to us as children.

So disengaging the issues that upset us from earlier in our lives we have to find a way to bond with our internal child, we then need to assist in rebuilding this part of us which will, in turn, help us to be rid of all that has been hindering us from moving on.

Connecting with your inner child may seem like something that may be hard or impossible to do, especially since they may be a part that has long been buried. It is a fairly easy exercise to do and can even be done right now. You will need about 20 minutes to complete this exercise. Here's what you do: find a quiet spot where you won't be disturbed and find pictures of you as a child if you think it may help.

Breathe in and loosen your clothing if you have to. Inhale deeply into your abdomen and exhale, repeat until you feel yourself getting relaxed; you may close your eyes and focus on getting less tense. Feel your forehead and head relax, let your face become relaxed and relax your shoulders. Allow your body to be limp and loose while you breathe slowly. Keep breathing slowly as you let all of your tension float away.

Now slowly count from 10 to 0 in your mind and try to think of a place from your childhood. The image doesn't have to be crystal clear right now but try to focus on exactly how you remember it and keep that image in mind. Imagine yourself as a child and imagine observing younger you; think about your clothes, expression, hair, etc. In your mind go and meet yourself, introduce yourself to you.

Chapter 1: How Does the Mind Work?

Your mind plays a critical role in helping you get healthy, get in shape, and stay that way. Your account is so vital that if you can't get your mind to cooperate with your body, you could be seriously undermining your chances of improving your overall health and wellbeing.

Often getting your head in line with your body is dependent on being able to make the most of your internal programming mechanism. In other words, what you tell yourself is vital to achieving anything you want. This self-talk can make, or break, your chances of becoming who you want to be.

For example, if you are continually telling yourself that you are not up to the task, that you are never going to make it, or that it is simply too hard to, then the chances of you not achieving your goals will be very slim. In contrast, if your self-talk is based upon your understanding of what it takes to be the best version of yourself, then the chances of you achieving anything that you want can explode through the roof. Best of all, you will give yourself a fighting chance when it comes to warding off any unwanted thoughts and feelings.

Also, it is vital to consider the fact that input from external sources can wreak havoc on your self-confidence and the way your mind process such data. You might get negative messages from people around you, or even attacks upon your choice of a healthy lifestyle. In some cases, attacks go to such extremes that some people stop talking to you, or decide not to hang out with you anymore, simply because you don't partake in eating or drinking binges.

These are people that you don't need in your life. It is best to surround yourself with like-minded people who will support you and help you in your endeavors. In doing so, you will be able to make better choices and stay on track.

Ultimately, you have the power to get on track and stay there. You don't need to depend on anything to help you make the most of your abilities to get in shape, drop some pounds and improve your overall health and wellbeing. Sure, it helps to be surrounded by

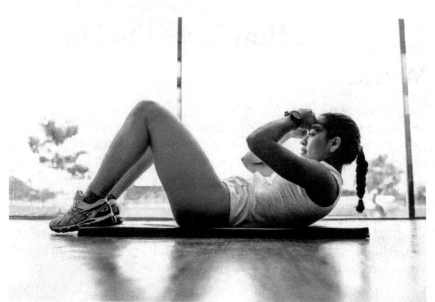

supportive friends and family. But in the end, you have everything you need to be successful.

Throughout this the discussion presented, we are going to be looking at how you can summon that inner willpower that you have to aid you in making the most of any changes that you need to make... and help them stick. After all, anyone can go on one of those crash diets. But what will help you truly become what you want to be is your desire and willingness to make things happen. That coupled with a robust methodology, such as the power of meditation, you will come to develop your winning formula. You can think that this isn't a cookie-cutter solution. This is the type of approach which you can build for yourself. That means that what you do, what you choose to accomplish, and the way that you decide to do it will be your own particular way of doing things. That will surely guarantee that what you do will be both successful and sustainable.

With that in your back pocket, you can feel confident about moving on to bigger and better things in your life. You won't have to worry about being successful ever again simply because you have already achieved the most critical goal in your life. Based on that, you can begin to feel comfortable in your skin. And there is nothing better than feeling good about yourself while making the best of your opportunity to achieve everything that you have always wanted to achieve.

Chapter 2: What is Hypnosis?

Many psychiatrists have long considered hypnosis as a decent and respectable therapy method and it has become one of the regular psychiatric practices along with being showcased in Hollywood movies and poor illusion shows. Despite the general consensus, hypnosis is not an illusion, but it is a serious medical treatment if it is applied appropriately. Its helpfulness is undeniable; however, it can also be hazardous. Why? Because in some regards, hypnosis is a kind of mind control technique. Furthermore, hypnosis is sometimes still recognized to be some mysterious phenomenon, or more 'rational' people simply view it as a trick. The 'enlightened' scientific version of the latter opinion claims that the hypnotized subject almost always tries to meet the expectations of the hypnotist; therefore, the hypnotic phenomena are nothing more than role-playing.

What is the truth about hypnosis?

What if hypnosis isn't just the tricky deception we see at shows? The truth is that hypnosis is closely connected to meditation. Hypnosis uses techniques of deep breathing and puts the subject into an incredibly powerful relaxed state in order to make them open to suggestions. This psychiatric technique does not apply the usage of a pendulum in front of a person's eyes, as is commonly believed. What it does is to create a relaxed atmosphere so that the patient can feel comfortable and trust in their therapist. The purpose is to be able to reach the patient at different conscious levels so that they can be more open to suggestions.

How did hypnosis originate?

Theories suggest that people may have used hypnosis as early as prehistoric times. The rites of worship and shamanism are partly explained by self-suggestion. It was presumably discovered accidentally through religious activities such as meditation, cult activities, and rituals. The first figures, most likely about hypnosis, have survived from ancient Egypt. The oldest description is on an Egyptian papyrus roll from 3766 BC: "Put your hand on the arm to relieve the pain and say that the pain has ceased." The Westcar papyrus preserved at the Neues Museum in Berlin reports that Jaya-manekh had persuaded a very wild lion to obey him. This source undoubtedly indicates that animal hypnosis was already known and practiced in Egypt. They may have known about hypnosis utilized with humans. Along with Jaya-manekh, Deda also used animal hypnosis, though he only presented his evidence using ducks, geese and an ox (Mongiovi, 2014).

The roots of what we now call hypnosis must be found at the end of the Middle Ages and in modern times.

In the sixteenth century, Paracelsus hypothesized about the devious relationship between celestial bodies and the human body. He considered it important to use various mineral medicines in addition to the proper magic spells. This laid the foundation for the theory of "mineral magnetism." Franz Anton Mesmer (1720-1815) adopted and continued the principle of magnetic effect. Through his group healings in a spectacular séance (reminiscent of the exorcism ceremony in its outward appearance), he became well-known for being the founder of the first hypnosis school. Nonetheless, in practice, verbal suggestion was lacking. He attributed therapeutic efficacy to the mysterious "magnetic fluid" that could be transmitted to the patient by hand movement ("magnetic passage") over the patient's body. He explained this with animated magnetism ('magnetismus animalis'; the magnetism of breathing, soul-like creatures) and placed magnets on the patients. Because of its popularity, hypnosis has long been called mesmerization (Rose, 2017).

Many others later criticized Mesmer. For example, Alfred Russel Wallace explained hypnosis with a phrenological map, and Friedrich Engels hypnotized a 12-year-old boy without a magnet. Mesmer was a pupil of the Marquis Armand-Marc-Jacques de Chastenet Puitureur (1721-1825). He initially accepted his master's theory, but his practice, unlike Mesmer's, lacked spectacular elements. His patients, who were subjected to verbal suggestions, behaved similarly to sleepwalkers and called their condition provocative somnambulism (Mongiovi, 2014).

If you've watched some of the old western movies, you may have noticed that alcohol was utilized as an anesthetic in operations. A few hundred years ago, if someone's arm had to be amputated, the patient would have been given a cheap whiskey for numbing purposes because they didn't have the luxury of using medicines like today. But alcohol wasn't the only anesthetic method. Hypnosis was also used for similar reasons to relieve pain in order to prevent subjects from entering neurogenic shock in the 1800s. If you really think about it, this was a very useful method. One of the best examples of the use of hypnosis in surgery is James Esdaile, a Scottish doctor who applied the method to more than 3000 patients in India with superior accomplishment (Spiegel, 2007).

In the 19th century, France took the lead in hypnosis research with centers such as Nancy (Ambroise-Auguste Liebeault, Hippolyte Bernheim) and Paris (Jean-Martin Charcot). Sigmund Freud visited Jean-Martin Charcot in Paris in 1885, observing Mesmer's method and trying it out for himself. This became the starting point for his studies on hysteria. He later abandoned this method and switched to free association. It is clear from his writings that he continued to deal with hypnosis. Oskar Vogt (1870-1959) and his student Johannes Heinrich Schultz (1884-1970) researched and developed autogenous training from German hypnosis. Later Klaus Thomas did research as well. The main researchers in America were Milton H. Erickson (indirect hypnosis), and Kroger and Dave Elman (authorial hypnosis). John Hartland is the best-known hypnotist in the UK. His book, the Dictionary of Medical and Dental Hypnosis, is still the official textbook for British hypnotists. Milton H. Erickson developed the method of hypnotherapy, from which several psychological techniques were improved.

Can anyone be hypnotized?

Hypnosis is an unpredictable state. You may be easily hypnotized, while it won't work for others. It is still a mystery to psychiatrists and neuroscientists how hypnosis works. The only thing we know is that it can work, but we don't have any idea how it works. A scientific study on the mechanism of hypnosis researched why some people are more responsive to hypnosis than others. As reported by the research, an individual's hypnotizability is more easily linked to brain function and the capability of connection. According to the study, the relationships between the left dorsolateral prefrontal cortex and the brain areas that treat the information are more effective than those of other subjects (Hoeft, Gabrieli, Whitfield-Gabrieli, Haas, Bammer, Menon, & Spiegel, 2013). Dr. Clifford N. Lazarus says that the individual must be willing and open to hypnosis; otherwise, it doesn't work: "Contrary to popular belief, people under hypnosis are in total control of themselves and would never do anything they would normally find highly objectionable" (Lazarus, 2013). It implies that if you don't want to be hypnotized, you can resist.

What occurs during hypnotism?

Imagine that you are watching an exciting action movie. A dangerous group chases the main character. The protagonist is trapped in a building, and the bad guys are waiting for him outside. You have been immersed in the movie when one of your family members asks you to give them a pillow. What do you do? I suppose you will take the pillow and give it to your relative without taking your eyes off the screen. When you are hypnotized, a similar scenario occurs. You focus on the matter intensely, and everything else becomes irrelevant. The greater the focus, the stronger the tendency to follow the suggestions of the therapist.

However, there is a tiny difference between the attention paid during a movie and in hypnosis. People who watch movies profoundly are more inclined not to reply to the questions they are asked; however, the opposite occurs during hypnosis. Why is that? Based on the observation of Freudian psychologists, this happens due to the difference between the phases of human awareness. They believe that there are three layers of human consciousness: preconsciousness, consciousness, and the unconscious level. These levels are depicted with an analogy. The level of consciousness that is compared to the visible part of an iceberg seeing it from the water surface represents the moments of our awareness about what's happening around us when we are awake (Cherry, 2019).

The iceberg's water level represents the level of preconsciousness and illustrates what we can't remember at the very moment but can recall if we want to. For instance, when you need to go somewhere that you have been before but don't remember the way, you will still find the right street. How is it possible? Because your preconsciousness level provides you with the necessary information to easily find the way you don't remember. You don't store this information in the level of consciousness. The part which is underwater and has the most massive volume is associated with the unconscious level in the iceberg analogy. We store fears, irrational and unacceptable desires, and deep convictions at the unconscious level. In order to bring them to the surface, we use hypnosis which can touch this level of our awareness. In the unconscious phase, right or wrong, moral or immoral don't exist because the filter system, which directs a person's ordinary life, is disabled, and our capacity for analyzing matters is discharged. In this level of consciousness, our deepest desires come true. However, unlike in a dream, our ability to perceive danger is still alert during hypnosis which means if the individual fears hypnosis or considers it dangerous, they won't allow the therapist to reach that phase of awareness (Journal Psyche, n. d.).

Can we really recall the hidden parts of our past under hypnosis?

Many therapists think that unsolved dilemmas or issues in the past are transmitted to the future, confusing people and producing psychological disorders. Therapists use the method of hypnosis to make their patients remember their past lives and release 'emotional baggage'. However, we need to know that memory is in an unstable form in the hypnotic subconscious. Therefore, hypnosis can cause a person to think that they are experiencing an event that hasn't occurred in real life. Hence, many experts reject the thesis that details are remembered, as they can be easily distorted. But it also means that we can alter our negative memories and convictions and exchange them with favorable ones (Thompson, n. d.).

Is hypnosis a biological phenomenon?

Research suggests that hypnosis has a biological aspect because of an electrical impulse between our brain cells. Cells send these impulses synchronously in groups and they don't isolate them. Also, various phases of consciousness have different frequencies (brain wave rhythm). If we acknowledge the electrical impulses as the language of the brain, we can pretend that different frequencies communicate at different speeds. These different speeds are called Alpha, Beta, Theta and Delta.

When we are asleep, the brain waves slow down and produce the so-called delta frequency waves. When it reveals relatively higher frequency vigilance, this is called beta frequency waves. Research has shown that brain waves are at theta frequency during hypnosis. In the theta frequency, there is both a level of subconscious awareness as well as a high concentration in sleep. It has been noticed that theta frequency occurs more frequently in the brains of people who are more susceptible to hypnosis.

Besides, some researchers claim that hypnotizability is inherited and strongly conditioned by the presence of specific genes (Adachi, Jensen, Lee, Miró, Osman, Tomé-Pires, 2016).

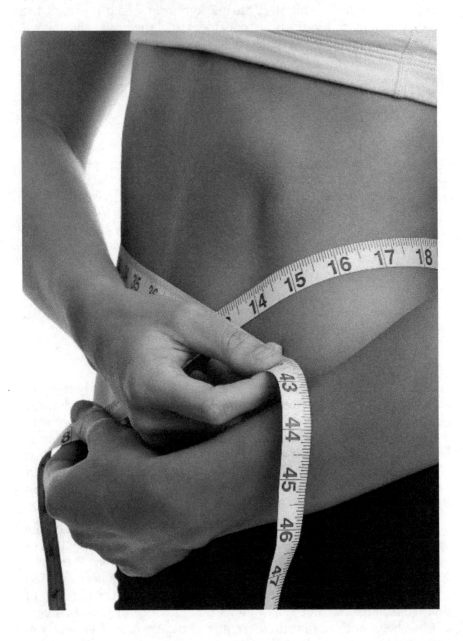

Chapter 3: How Hypnosis Can Help You Lose Weight

Losing weight with hypnosis works just like any other change with hypnosis will. However, it is important to understand the step-by-step process so that you know exactly what to expect during your weight loss journey with the support of hypnosis. In general, there are about seven steps that are involved with weight loss using hypnosis. The first step is when you decide to change; the second step involves your sessions; the third and fourth are your changed mindset and behaviors, the fifth step involves your regressions, the sixth is your management routines, and the seventh is your lasting change. To give you a better idea of what each of these parts of your journey looks like, let's explore them in greater detail below.

In your first step toward achieving weight loss with hypnosis, you have decided that you desire change and that you are willing to try hypnosis as a way to change your approach to weight loss. At this point, you are aware of the fact that you want to lose weight, and you have been shown the possibility of losing weight through hypnosis. You may find yourself feeling curious, open to trying something new, and a little bit skeptical as to whether or not this is actually going to work for you. You may also be feeling frustrated, overwhelmed, or even defeated by the lack of success you have seen using other weight loss methods, which may be what lead you to seek out hypnosis in the first place. At this stage, the best thing you can do is practice keeping an open and curious mind, as this is how you can set yourself up for success when it comes to your actual hypnosis sessions.

Your sessions account for stage two of the process. Technically, you are going to move from stage two through to stage five several times over before you officially move into stage six. Your sessions are the stage where you actually engage in hypnosis, nothing more and nothing less. During your sessions, you need to maintain your open mind and stay focused on how hypnosis can help you. If you are struggling to stay open-minded or are still skeptical about how this might work, you can consider switching from absolute confidence that it will help to have a curiosity about how it might help instead.

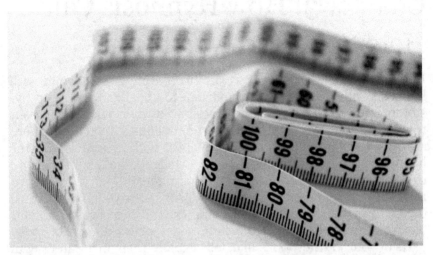

Following your sessions, you are first going to experience a changed mindset. This is where you start to feel far more confident in your ability to lose weight and in your ability to keep the weight off. At first, your mindset may still be shadowed by doubt, but as you continue to use hypnosis and see your results, you will realize that it is entirely possible for you to create success with hypnosis. As these pieces of evidence start to show up in your own life, you will find your hypnosis sessions becoming even more powerful and even more successful.

In addition to a changed mindset, you are going to start to see changed behaviors. They may be smaller at first, but you will find that they increase over time until they reach the point where your behaviors reflect exactly the lifestyle you have been aiming to have. The best part about these changed behaviors is that they will not feel forced, nor will they feel like you have had to encourage yourself to get here: your changed mindset will make these changed behaviors incredibly easy for you to choose. As you continue working on your hypnosis and experiencing your changed mind, you will find that your behavioral changes grow more significant and more effortless every single time.

Following your hypnosis and your experiences with changed mindset and behaviors, you are likely going to experience regression periods. Regression periods are characterized by periods of time where you begin to engage in your old mindset and behavior once again. This happens because you have experienced this old mindset and behavioral patterns so many times over that they continue to have deep roots in your subconscious mind. The more you uproot them and reinforce your new behaviors with consistent hypnosis sessions, the more success you will have in eliminating these old behaviors and replacing them entirely with new ones. Anytime you experience the beginning of a regression period; you should set aside some time to engage in a hypnosis session to help you shift your mindset back into the state that you want and need it to be in.

Your management routines account for the sixth step, and they come into place after you have effectively experienced a significant and lasting change from your hypnosis practices. At this point, you are not going to need to schedule as frequent of hypnosis sessions because you are experiencing such significant changes in your mindset. However, you may still want to do hypnosis sessions on a fairly consistent basis to ensure that your mindset remains changed and that you do not revert into old patterns. Sometimes, it can take up to 3-6 months or longer with these consistent management routine hypnosis sessions to maintain your changes and prevent you from experiencing a significant regression in your mindset and behavior.

The final step in your hypnosis journey is going to be the step where you come upon lasting changes. At this point, you are unlikely to need to schedule hypnosis sessions any longer. You should not need to rely on hypnosis at all to change your mindset because you have experienced such significant changes already, and you no longer find yourself regressing into old behaviors. With that being said, you may find that from time to time, you need to have a hypnosis session just to maintain your changes, particularly when an unexpected trigger may arise that may cause you to want to regress your behaviors. These unexpected changes can happen for years following your successful changes, so staying on top of them and relying on your healthy coping method of hypnosis is important as it will prevent you from experiencing a significant regression later in life.

Using Hypnosis to Encourage Healthy Eating and Discourage Unhealthy Eating

As you go through using hypnosis to support you with weight loss, there are a few ways that you are going to do so. One of the ways is, obviously, to focus on weight loss itself. Another way, however, is to focus on topics surrounding weight loss. For example, you can use hypnosis to help you encourage yourself to eat healthy while also helping discourage yourself from unhealthy eating. Effective hypnosis sessions can help you bust cravings for foods that are going to sabotage your success while also helping you feel more drawn to making choices that are going to help you effectively lose weight.

Many people will use hypnosis as a way to change their cravings, improve their metabolism, and even help themselves acquire a taste for eating healthier foods. You may also use this to help encourage you to develop the motivation and energy to actually prepare healthier foods and eat them so that you are more likely to have these healthier options available for you. If cultivating the motivation for preparing and eating healthy foods has been problematic for you, this type of hypnosis focus can be incredibly helpful.

Using Hypnosis to Encourage Healthy Lifestyle Changes

In addition to helping you encourage yourself to eat healthier while discouraging yourself from eating unhealthy foods, you can also use hypnosis to help encourage you to make healthy lifestyle changes. This can support you with everything from exercising more frequently to picking up more active hobbies that support your wellbeing in general.

You may also use this to help you eliminate hobbies or experiences from your life that may encourage unhealthy dietary habits in the first place. For example, if you tend to binge eat when you are stressed out, you might use hypnosis to help you navigate stress more effectively so that you are less likely to binge eat when you are feeling stressed out. If you tend to eat when you are feeling emotional or bored, you can use hypnosis to help you change those behaviors, too.

Hypnosis can be used to change virtually any area of your life that motivates you to eat unhealthily or otherwise neglect self-care to the point where you are sabotaging yourself from healthy weight loss. It truly is an incredibly versatile practice that you can rely on that will help you with weight loss, as well as help you with creating a healthier lifestyle in general. With hypnosis, there are countless ways that you can improve the quality of your life, making it an incredibly helpful practice for you to rely on.

The Benefits of Hypnotherapy for Weight Loss

It is hard to pinpoint the single best benefit that comes from using hypnosis as a way to engage in weight loss. Hypnosis is a natural, lasting, and deeply impactful weight loss habit that you can use to completely change the way you approach weight loss, and food in general, for the rest of your life.

With hypnosis, you are not ingesting anything that results in hypnosis working. Instead, you are simply listening to guided hypnosis meditations that help you transform the way your subconscious mind works. As you change the way your subconscious mind works, you will find yourself not even having cravings or unhealthy food urges in the first place. This means no more fighting against your desires, yo-yo dieting, "falling off the wagon," or experiencing any inner conflict around your eating patterns, or your weight loss exercises that are helping you lose the weight. Instead, you will begin to have an entirely new mindset and perspective around weight loss that leads to you having more success in losing weight and keeping it off for good.

In addition to hypnosis itself being effective, you can also combine hypnosis with any other weight loss strategy you are using. Changed dietary behaviors, exercise routines, any medications you may be taking with the advisement of your medical practitioner, and any other weight loss practices you may be engaging in can all safely be done with hypnosis. By including hypnosis in your existing weight loss routines, you can improve your effectiveness and rapidly increase the success you experience in your weight loss patterns.

Finally, hypnosis can be beneficial for many things beyond weight loss. One of the side effects that you will probably notice once you start using hypnosis to help change your weight loss experience is that you also experience a boost in your confidence, self-esteem, and general feelings of positivity. Many people who use hypnosis on a regular basis find themselves feeling more positive and in better spirits in general. This means that not only will you lose weight, but you will also feel incredible and will have a happy and positive mood as well.

Chapter 4: What is Self-Hypnosis?

If you can afford to undergo a series of hypnotherapy sessions with a specialist, you may do so. This is ideal as you will work with a professional who can guide you through the treatment and will also provide you with valuable advice on nutrition and exercises.

Clinical Hypnotherapy

When first meeting with a therapist, they start by explaining to you the type of hypnotherapy he or she is using. Then you will discuss your personal goals so the therapist can better understand your motivations.

The formal session will start with your therapist, speaking in a gentle and soothing voice. This will help you relax and feel safe during the entire therapy.

Once your mind is more receptive, the therapist will start suggesting ways that can help you modify your exercise or eating habits as well as other ways to help you reach your weight loss goals.

Specific words or repetition of particular phrases can help you at this stage. The therapist may also help you in visualizing the body image you want, which is one effective technique in hypnotherapy.

To end the session, the therapist will bring you out from the hypnotic stage, and you will start to be more alert. Your personal goals will influence the duration of the hypnotherapy sessions as well as the number of total sessions that you may need. Most people begin to see results in as few as two to four sessions.

DIY Hypnotherapy

If you are not comfortable working with a professional hypnotherapist or you can't afford the sessions, you can choose to perform self-hypnosis. While this is not as effective as the sessions under a professional, you can still try it and see if it can help you with your weight loss goals.

HERE ARE THE STEPS IF YOU WISH TO PRACTICE SELF-HYPNOSIS:

Believe in the power of hypnotism. Remember, this alternative treatment requires the person to be open and willing.

It will not work for you if your mind is already set against it.

Find a comfortable and quiet room to practice hypnotherapy. Ideally, you should find a place that is free from noise and where no one can disturb you. Wear loose clothes and set relaxing music to help in setting up the mood.

Find a focal point. Choose an object in a room that you can focus on. Use your concentration on this object so you can start clearing your mind of all thoughts.

Breathe deeply. Start with five deep breaths, inhaling through your nose and exhaling through your mouth.

Close your eyes. Think about your eyelids becoming heavy and just let them close slowly.

Imagine that all stress and tension are coming out of your body. Let this feeling move down from your head, to your shoulders, to your chest, to your arms, to your stomach, to your legs, and finally to your feet.

Clear your mind. When you are relaxed, your account must be clear, and you can initiate the process of self-hypnotism.

Visualize a pendulum. In your mind, picture a moving swing. The movement of the pendulum is popular imagery used in hypnotism to encourage focus.

Start visualizing your ideal body image and size. This should help you instill in your subconscious the importance of a healthy diet and exercise.

Suggest to yourself to avoid unhealthy food and start exercising regularly. You can use a particular mantra such as "I will exercise at least three times a week. Unhealthy food will make me sick."

Wake up. Once you have achieved what you want during hypnosis, you must wake yourself. Start by counting back from one to 10 and wake up when you reach 10.

Remember, a healthy diet doesn't mean that you have to reduce your food intake significantly. Just cut your consumption of food that is not healthy for you. Never hypnotize yourself out of eating. Only suggest to yourself to eat less of the food that you know is just making you fat.

Chapter 5: Hypnosis and Weight Loss

Hypnosis plays a vital role in medicinal solutions. In modern-day society, it is recommended for treating many different conditions, including obesity or weight loss in individuals who are overweight. It also serves patients who have undergone surgery exceptionally well, mainly if they are restricted from exercising after surgery. Given that it is the perfect option for losing weight, it is additionally helpful to anyone who is disabled or recovering from an injury.

Once you understand the practice and how it is conducted, you will find that everything makes sense. Hypnosis works for weight loss because of the relationship between our minds and bodies. Without proper communication being relayed from our minds to our bodies, we would not be able to function correctly. Since hypnosis allows the brain to adopt new ideas and habits, it can help push anyone in the right direction and could potentially improve our quality of living.

Adopting new habits can help eliminate fear, improve confidence, and inspire you to maintain persistence and a sense of motivation on your weight loss journey. Since two of the most significant issue's society faces today are media-based influences and a lack of motivation, you can quickly solve any problems related by merely correcting your mind.

Correcting your mind is an entirely different mission on its own, or without hypnosis, that is. It is a challenge that most will get frustrated. Nobody wants to deal with themselves. Although that may be true, perhaps one of the best lessons hypnosis teaches you is the significance of spending time focusing on your intentions. Daily practicing of hypnosis includes focusing on specific ideas. Once these ideas are normalized in your daily routine and life, you will find it easier to cope with struggles and ultimately break bad habits, which is the ultimate goal.

In reality, it takes 21 consecutive days to break a bad habit, but only if a person remains persistent, integrating both a conscious and consistent effort to quit or rectify a practice. It takes the same amount of time to adopt a new healthy habit. With hypnosis, it can take up to three months to either break a bad habit or form a

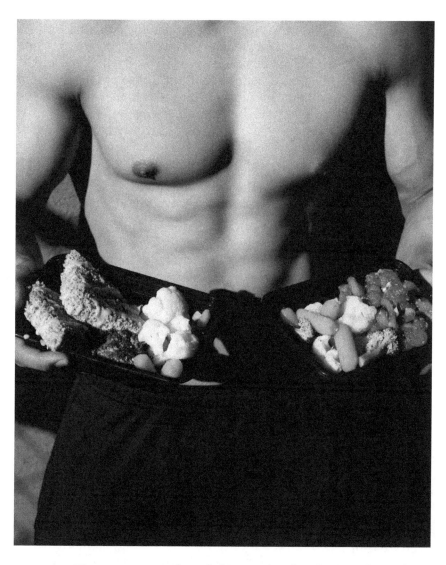

new one. However, even though hypnosis takes longer, it tends to work far more effectively than just forcing yourself to do something you don't want to do.

Our brains are robust operating systems that can be fooled under the right circumstances. Hypnosis has been proven to be useful for breaking habits and adopting new ones due to its powerful effect on the mind. It can be measured in the same line of consistency and power as affirmations. Now, many would argue that hypnosis is unnecessary and that completing a 90-day practice of hypnotherapy to change habits for weight loss is a complete waste of time. However, when you think about someone who needs to lose weight but can't seem to do it, then you might start reconsidering it as a helpful solution to the problem. It's no secret that the human brain requires far more than a little push or single affirmation to thrive. Looking at motivational video clips and reading quotes every day is great, but is it helping you to move further than from A to B?

It's true that today, we are faced with a sense of rushing through life. Asking an obese or unhealthy individual why they gained weight, there's a certainty that you'll receive similar answers.

Could it be that no one has time to, for instance, cook or prep healthy meals, visit the gym or move their bodies? Apart from making up excuses as to why you can't do something, there's actual evidence hidden in the reasons why we sell ourselves short and opt for the easy way out.

Could it be that the majority of individuals have just become lazy?

Regardless of your excuses, reasons or inabilities, hypnosis debunks the idea that you have to go all out to get healthier. Losing weight to improve your physical appearance has always been a challenge, and although there is no easy way out, daily persistence and 10 to 60 minutes a day of practice could help you to lose weight. Not just that, but it can also restructure your brain and help you to develop better habits, which will guide you in experiencing a much more positive and sustainable means of living.

Regardless of the practice or routine, you follow at the end of the day, the principle of losing weight always remains the same. You have to follow a balanced diet in proportion with a sustainable exercise routine.

By not doing so is where most people tend to go wrong with their weight loss journeys. It doesn't matter whether it's a diet supplement, weight loss tea, or even hypnosis. Your diet and exercise routine still play an increasingly important role in losing weight and will be the number one factor that will help you to obtain permanent results. There's a lot of truth in the advice given that there aren't any quick fixes to help you lose weight faster than what's recommended. Usually, anything that promotes standard weight loss, which is generally about two to five pounds a week, depending on your current Body Mass Index (BMI), works no matter what it is. The trick to losing weight doesn't necessarily lie in what you do, but instead in how you do it.

When people start with hypnosis, they may be very likely to quit after a few days or weeks, as it may not seem useful or it isn't leading to any noticeable results.

Nevertheless, if you remain consistent with it, eat a balanced diet instead of crash dieting, and follow a simple exercise routine, then you will find that it has a lot more to offer you than just weight loss. Even though weight loss is the ultimate goal, it's essential to keep in mind that lasting results don't occur overnight. There are no quick fixes, especially with hypnosis.

Adopting the practice, you will discover many benefits, yet two of the most important ones are healing and learning how to activate the fat burning process inside of your body.

Hypnosis is not a diet, nor is it a fast track method to get you where you want to go. Instead, it is a tool used to help individuals reach their goals by implementing proper habits. These habits can help you achieve results by focusing on appropriate diet and exercise. Since psychological issues influence most weight-related issues, hypnosis acts as the perfect tool, laying a foundation for a healthy mind.

Hypnosis is not a type of mind control, yet it is designed to alter your mind by shifting your feelings toward liking something that you might have hated before, such as exercise or eating a balanced diet. The same goes for quitting sugar or binge eating. Hypnosis identifies the root of the issues you may be dealing with and works by rectifying it accordingly. Given that it changes your thought pattern, you may also experience a much calmer and relaxed approach to everything you do.

Hypnosis works by maintaining changes made in mind because of neuroplasticity. Consistent hypnotherapy sessions create new patterns in the brain that result in the creation of new habits. Since consistency is the number one key to losing weight, it acts as a solution to overcome barriers in your mind, which is something the majority of individuals struggle. Hypnosis can also provide you with many techniques to meet different goals, such as gastric band hypnosis, which works by limiting eating habits, causing you to refrain from overeating.

Chapter 6: The Power of Affirmations

Today is another day. Today is a day for you to start making a euphoric, satisfying life. Today is the day to begin to discharge every one of your impediments. Today is the day for you to get familiar with the privileged insights of life. You can transform yourself into improving things. You, as of now, include the devices inside you to do as such. These devices are your considerations and your convictions.

What Are Positive Affirmations?

For those of you who aren't acquainted with the advantages of positive affirmations, I'd prefer to clarify a little about them. A statement is genuinely anything you state or think. A great deal of what we typically report and believe is very harmful and doesn't make great encounters for us. We need to retrain our reasoning and to talk into positive examples if we need to change us completely.

An affirmation opens the entryway. It's a starting point on the way to change. When I talk about doing affirmations, I mean deliberately picking words that will either help take out something from your life or help make something new in your life.

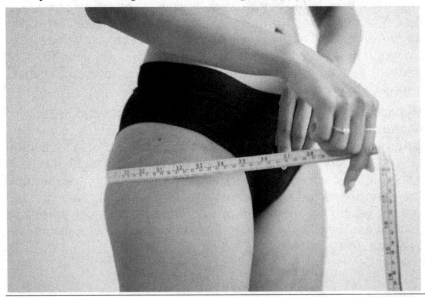

Each idea you think and each word you express is an affirmation. The entirety of our self-talk, our interior exchange, is a flood of oaths. You're utilizing statements each second, whether you know it or not. You're insisting and making your background with each word and thought.

Your convictions are just routine reasoning examples that you learned as a youngster. The vast numbers of them work very well for you. Different beliefs might be restricting your capacity to make the very things you state you need. What you need and what you trust your merit might be unusual. You have to focus on your contemplations with the goal that you can start to dispose of the ones making encounters you don't need in your life.

It would help if you understood that each grievance is an affirmation of something you figure you don't need in your life. Each time you blow up, you're asserting that you need more annoyance in your life. Each time you feel like a casualty, you're confirming that you need to keep on feeling like a casualty. If you believe that you think that life isn't giving you what you need in your reality, at that point, it's sure that you will never have the treats that experience provides for others that is until you change how you think and talk.

You're not a terrible individual for intuition, how you do. You've quite recently never figured out how to think and talk. Individuals all through the world are quite recently starting to discover that our contemplations make our encounters. Your folks most likely didn't have the foggiest idea about this, so they couldn't in any way, shape, or form instruct it to you. They showed you what to look like at life in the manner that their folks told them. So, no one isn't right. In any case, it's the ideal opportunity for us all to wake up and start to deliberately make our lives in a manner that satisfies and bolsters us. You can do it. I can do it. We, as a whole, can do it, we need to figure out how. So how about we get to it?

I'll talk about affirmations as a rule, and afterwards, I'll get too specific everyday issues and tell you the best way to roll out positive improvements in your wellbeing, your funds, your affection life, etc. Once you figure out how to utilize affirmations, at that point, you can apply the standards in all circumstances. A few people say that "affirmations don't work" (which is an affirmation in itself) when what they mean is that they don't have a clue how to utilize them accurately. Some of the time, individuals will say their affirmations once per day and gripe the remainder of the time. It will require some investment for affirmations to work if they're done that way. The grumbling affirmations will consistently win, because there is a higher amount of them, and they're generally said with extraordinary inclination.

In any case, saying affirmations is just a piece of the procedure. What you wrap up of the day and night is significantly progressively significant. The key to having your statements work rapidly and reliably is to set up air for them to develop in. Affirmations resemble seeds planted in soil: poor soil, poor development. Fertile soil, bottomless event. The more you decide to think contemplations that cause you to feel great, the faster the affirmations work.

So, think upbeat musings, it's that straightforward. What's more, it is feasible. How you decide to believe at present is only a decision. You may not understand it since you've thought along these lines for such a long time, yet it truly is a decision. Presently, today, this second, you can decide to change your reasoning. Your life won't pivot for the time being. Yet, in case you're reliable and settle on the decision regularly to think considerations that cause you to feel great, you'll unquestionably roll out positive improvements in each part of your life.

Positive Affirmations and How to Use Them

Positive affirmations are positive articulations that depict an ideal circumstance, propensity, or objective that you need to accomplish. Rehashing regularly these positive explanations, influences the psyche brain profoundly, and triggers it without hesitation, to bring what you are reworking into the real world.

The demonstration of rehashing the affirmations, intellectually or so anyone might hear, inspires the individual reworking them, builds the desire and inspiration, and pulls in open doors for development and achievement.

This demonstration likewise programs the psyche to act as per the rehashed words, setting off the inner mind-brain to take a shot at one's sake, to offer the positive expressions materialize.

Affirmations are extremely valuable for building new propensities, rolling out positive improvements throughout one's life, and for accomplishing objectives.

Affirmations help in weight misfortune, getting progressively engaged, concentrating better, changing propensities, and accomplishing dreams.

They can be helpful in sports, in business, improving one's wellbeing, weight training, and in numerous different zones.

These positive articulations influence in a proper manner, the body, the brain, and one's sentiments

Rehashing affirmations is very reasonable. Despite this, a lot of people do not know about this truth. Individuals, for the most part, restate negative statements, not positive ones. This is called negative self-talk.

On the off chance that you have been disclosing to yourself how miserable you can't contemplate, need more cash, or how troublesome life is, you have been rehashing negative affirmations.

Along these lines, you make more challenges and more issues, since you are concentrating on the problems, and in this way, expanding them, rather than concentrating on the arrangements.

A great many people rehash in their psyches pessimistic words and proclamations concerning the contrary circumstances and occasions in their lives, and therefore, make progressively bothersome circumstances.

Words work in two different ways, to assemble or obliterate. It is how we use them that decides if they will bring tremendous or destructive outcomes.

Affirmations in Modern Times

It is said that the French analyst and drug specialist Emile Coue is the individual who carried this subject to the open's consideration in the mid-twentieth century.

Emile Coue saw that when he told his patients how viable an elixir was, the outcomes were superior to if he didn't utter a word. He understood that musings that consume our psyches become a reality and that rehashing concepts and considerations is a sort of autosuggestion.

Emile Coue is associated with his acclaimed proclamation, "Consistently, all around, I am showing signs of improvement and better."

Later in the twentieth century, this was Louise Hay, who concentrated on this point and called autosuggestion affirmations.

Chapter 7: 100 Positive Affirmations for Weight Loss

George taught Bonnie a hundred useful positive affirmations for weight loss and to keep her motivated. She chose the ones that she wanted to build in her program and used them every day. Bonnie was losing weight very slowly, which bothered her very much. She thought she was going in the wrong direction and was about to give up, but George told her not to worry because it was a completely natural speed. It takes time for the subconscious to collate all the information and start working according to her conscious will. Besides, her body remembered the fast weight loss, but her subconscious remembered her emotional damage, and now it is trying to prevent it. In reality, after some months of hard work, she started to see the desired results. She weighed 74 kilos (163 lbs.).

According to dietitians, the success of dieting is greatly influenced by how people talk about lifestyle changes for others and themselves.

The use of "I should," or "I must" is to avoid whenever possible. Anyone who says, "I shouldn't eat French fries," or "I have to get a bite of chocolate" will feel that they have no control over the events. Instead, if you say "I prefer" to leave the food, you will feel more power and less guilt. The term "dieting" should be avoided. Proper nutrition is a permanent lifestyle change. For example, the correct wording is, "I've changed my eating habits" or "I'm eating healthier."

Diets are fattening. Why?

The body needs fat. Our body wants to live, so it stores fat. Removing this amount of fat from the body is not an easy task as the body protects against weight loss. During starvation, our bodies switch to a 'saving flame', burning fewer calories to avoid starving. Those who are starting to lose weight are usually optimistic, as, during the first week, they may experience 1-3 kg (2-7 lbs.) Of weight loss, which validates their efforts and suffering. Their body, however, has deceived them very well because it actually does not want to break down fat. Instead, it begins to break down muscle tissue. At the beginning of dieting, our bodies burn sugar and protein, not fat. Burned sugar removes a lot of water out of the body; that's why we experience amazing results on the scale. It should take about seven days for our body to switch to fat burning. Then our body's alarm bell rings. Most diets have a sad end: reducing your metabolic rate to a lower level—meaning, that if you only eat a little more afterwards, you regain all the weight you have lost previously. After dieting, the body will make special efforts to store fat for the next impending famine. What to do to prevent such a situation?

We must understand what our soul needs. Those who really desire to have success must first and foremost change their spiritual foundation. It is important to pamper our souls during a period of weight loss. All overweight people tend to rag on themselves for eating forbidden food, "I overate again. My willpower is so weak!" If you have ever tried to lose weight, you know these thoughts very well.

Imagine a person very close to you who has gone through a difficult time while making mistakes from time to time. Are we going to scold or try to help and motivate them? If we really love them, we will instead comfort them and try to convince them to continue. No one tells their best friend that they are weak, ugly, or bad, just because they are struggling with their weight. If you wouldn't say it to your friend, don't do so to yourself either! Let us be aware of this: during weight loss, our soul needs peace and support. Realistic thinking is more useful than disaster theory. If you are generally a healthy consumer, eat some goodies sometimes because of its delicious taste and to pamper your soul.

I'll give you a list of a hundred positive affirmations you can use to reinforce your weight loss. I'll divide them into main categories based on the most typical situations for which you would need confirmation. You can repeat all of them whenever you need to, but you can also choose the ones that are more suitable for your circumstances. If you prefer to listen to them during meditation, you can record them with a piece of sweet relaxing music in the background.

General affirmations to reinforce your wellbeing:

1. I'm grateful that I woke up today. Thank you for making me happy today.

2. Today is a perfect day. I meet nice and helpful people, whom I treat kindly.

3. Every new day is for me. I live to make myself feel good. Today

I just pick good thoughts for myself.

4. Something wonderful is happening to me today.

5. I feel good.

6. I am calm, energetic and cheerful.

7. My organs are healthy.

8. I am satisfied and balanced.

9. I live in peace and understanding with everyone.

10. I listen to others with patience.

11. In every situation, I find the good.

12. I accept and respect myself and my fellow human beings.

13. I trust myself; I trust my inner wisdom.

Do you often scold yourself? Then repeat the following affirmations frequently:

14. I forgive myself.

15. I'm good to myself.

16. I motivate myself over and over again.

17. I'm doing my job well.

18. I care about myself.

19. I am doing my best.

20. I am proud of myself for my achievements.

21. I am aware that sometimes I have to pamper my soul.

22. I remember that I did a great job this week.

23. I deserved this small piece of candy.

24. I let go of the feeling of guilt.

25. I release the blame.

26. Everyone is imperfect. I accept that I am too.

If you feel pain when you choose to avoid delicious food, then you need to motivate yourself with affirmations such as:

27. I am motivated and persistent.

28. I control my life and my weight.

29. I'm ready to change my life.

30. Changes make me feel better.

31. I follow my diet with joy and cheerfulness.

32. I am aware of my amazing capacities.

33. I am grateful for my opportunities.

34. Today I'm excited to start a new diet.

35. I always keep in mind my goals.

36. I imagine myself slim and beautiful.

37. Today I am happy to have the opportunity to do what I have long been postponing.

38. I possess the energy and will to go through my diet.

39. I prefer to lose weight instead of wasting time on momentary pleasures.

Here you can find affirmations that help you to change harmful convictions and blockages:

40. I see my progress every day.

41. I listen to my body's messages.

42. I'm taking care of my health.

43. I eat healthy food.

44. I love who I am.

45. I love how life supports me.

46. A good parking space, coffee, conversation. It's all for me today.

47. It feels good to be awake because I can live in peace, health, love.

48. I'm grateful that I woke up. I take a deep breath of peace and tranquility.

49. I love my body. I love being served by me.

50. I eat by tasting every flavor of the food.

51. I am aware of the benefits of healthy food.

52. I enjoy eating healthy food and being fitter every day.

53. I feel energetic because I eat well.

Many people are struggling with being overweight because they don't move enough. The very root of this issue can be a refusal to do exercises due to negative biases in our minds.

We can overcome these beliefs by repeating the following affirmations:

54. I like moving because it helps my body burn fat.

55. Each time I exercise, I am getting closer to having a beautiful, tight shapely body.

56. It's a very uplifting feeling of being able to climb up to 100 steps without stopping.

57. It's easier to have an excellent quality of life if I move.

58. I like the feeling of returning to my home tired but happy after a long winter walk.

59. Physical exercises help me have a longer life.

60. I am proud to have better fitness and agility.

61. I feel happier thanks to the happiness hormone produced by exercise.

62. I feel full thanks to the enzymes that produce a sense of fullness during physical exercises.

63. I am aware even after exercise, my muscles continue to burn fat, and so I lose weight while resting.

64. I feel more energetic after exercises.

65. My goal is to lose weight; therefore, I exercise.

66. I am motivated to exercise every day.

67. I lose weight while I exercise.

Now, I am going to give you a list of generic affirmations that you can build in your program:

68. I'm glad I'm who I am.

69. Today, I read articles and watch movies that make me feel positive about my diet progress.

70. I love it when I'm happy.

71. I take a deep breath and exhale my fears.

72. Today I do not want to prove my truth, but I want to be happy.

73. I am strong and healthy. I'm fine, and I'm getting better.

74. I am happy today because whatever I do, I find joy in it.

75. I pay attention to what I can become.

76. I love myself and am helpful to others.

77. I accept what I cannot change.

78. I am happy that I can eat healthy food.

79. I am happy that I have been changing my life with my new healthy lifestyle.

80. Today I do not compare myself to others.

81. I accept and support who I am and turn to myself with love.

82. Today I can do anything for my improvement.

83. I'm fine. I'm happy for life. I love who I am. I'm strong and confident.

84. I am calm and satisfied.

85. Today is perfect for me to exercise and to be healthy.

86. I have decided to lose weight, and I am strong enough to follow my will.

87. I love myself, so I want to lose weight.

88. I am proud of myself because I follow my diet program.

89. I see how much stronger I am.

90. I know that I can do it.

91. It is not my past, but my present that defines me.

92. I am grateful for my life.

93. I am grateful for my body because it collaborates well with me.

94. Eating healthy foods supports me to get the best nutrients I need to be in the best shape.

95. I eat only healthy foods, and I avoid processed foods.

96. I can achieve my weight loss goals.

97. All cells in my body are fit and healthy, and so am I.

98. I enjoy staying healthy and sustaining my ideal weight.

99. I feel that my body is losing weight right now.

100. I care about my body by exercising every day.

Chapter 8: How to Practice Every Day

Exercise Regularly

Exercise is good for human health in many ways, regardless of what you choose to do.

Although the DASH diet focuses on food choices, there is no denying that regular and varied exercise represents an essential component of a healthy lifestyle and one that can confer additional benefits.

With that said, the CDC identifies moderate-intensity aerobic activity that totals 120 to 150 minutes weekly, in combination with two additional weekly days of muscular resistance training, as an ideal combination to confer numerous health benefits to adults. Per the CDC, these benefits include the following:

Better weight management: When combined with dietary modification, regular physical activity plays a role in supporting or enhancing weight-management efforts. Regular exercise is a great way to expend calories on top of any dietary changes you will be making on this program.

Reduced risk for cardiovascular disease: A reduction in blood pressure is a well-recognized benefit of regular physical activity, which ultimately contributes to a reduced risk of cardiovascular disease.

Reduced risk of type 2 diabetes: Regular physical activity is known to improve blood glucose control and insulin sensitivity.

Improved mood: Regular physical activity is associated with improvements in mood and reductions in anxiety owing to how exercise positively influences the biochemistry of the human brain by releasing hormones and affecting neurotransmitters.

Better sleep: Those who exercise more regularly tend to sleep better than those who don't, which may be partly owing to the reductions in stress and anxiety that often occur in those who exercise regularly.

Stronger bones and muscles: Combining cardiovascular and resistance training confers severe benefits to both your bones and your muscles, which keep your body functioning at a high level as

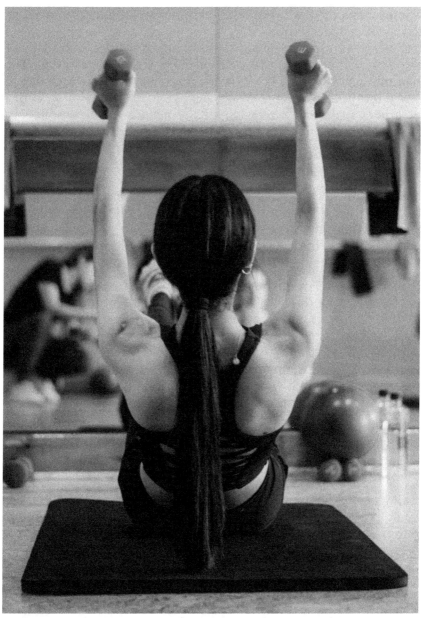

you age.

A longer life span: Those who exercise regularly tend to enjoy a lower risk of chronic disease and a longer life span.

As you will see in the 28-day plan, your recommended exercise totals will meet by exercising four out of the seven days a week.

The exercise days will break up as follows: All four of the active days will include aerobic exercise for 30 minutes. As a beginner, I encourage you to start slowly and build up to four days. Two of the four active days will also include strength training. The bottom line is that you don't have to exercise for hours each day to enjoy the health benefits of physical activity. Our goal with this plan is to make the health benefits of exercise as accessible and attainable as possible for those who are ready and willing to give it a try.

Getting the Most Out of Your Workouts

Just as with healthy eating strategies, there are certain essential things to keep in mind about physical activity that will help support your long-term success. Let's take a look at a few crucial considerations that will help you get the most out of your workouts:

Rest days: Even though we haven't even started, I'm going to preach the importance of proper rest. Don't forget that you are taking part in this journey to improve your health for the long term, not to burn yourself out in 28 days. Although some of you with more experience with exercise may feel confident going above and beyond, my best advice for the majority of those reading is to listen to your body and take days off to minimize the risk of injury and burnout.

Stretching life: Stretching is a great way to prevent injury and keep your pain-free both during workouts and daily. Whether it's a planned activity after an exercise or through additional means such as yoga, stretching is beneficial in many ways.

Enjoyment: There is no right or wrong style of exercise. You are being provided with a different plan that emphasizes a variety of different cardiovascular and resistance training exercises. If there are certain activities within these groups that you don't enjoy, it's okay not to do them. Your ability to stick with regular physical activity in the long term will depend on finding a style of exercise that you enjoy.

Your limits: Physical activity is right for you, and it should be fun, too. It's up to you to keep it that way. While it is essential to challenge yourself, don't risk injury by taking things too far too fast.

Your progress: Although this is not an absolute requirement, some of you reading may find joy and fulfilment through tracking your exercise progress and striving toward a longer duration, more repetitions, and so on. If you are the type who enjoys a competitive edge, it may be fun to find a buddy to exercise and progress with.

Warm-ups: Last but certainly not least, your exercise routine will benefit significantly from a proper warm-up routine, which includes starting slowly or doing exercises similar to the ones included in your workout, but at a lower intensity.

Set a Routine

The exercise part of the DASH plan was developed with CDC exercise recommendations in mind to support your best health. For some, the 28-day policy may seem like a lot; for others, it may not seem like that much. If we look at any exercise routine from a very general perspective, there are at least three broad categories to be aware of.

Strength training: This involves utilizing your muscles against some form of counterweight, which may be your own body or dumbbells. These types of activities alter your resting metabolic rate by supporting the development of muscle while also strengthening your bones.

Aerobic exercise: Also known as a cardiovascular activity, these are the quintessential exercises such as jogging or running that involve getting your body moving and getting your heart rate up.

Mobility, flexibility, and balance: Stretching after workouts or even devoting your exercise time on one day a week to stretching or yoga is a great way to maintain mobility and prevent injury in the long term.

This routine recommends involving a combination of both cardiovascular and resistance training.

You will be provided with a wide array of options to choose from to accommodate a diverse exercise routine.

My best recommendation is to settle on the types of exercises that offer a balance between enjoyment and challenge. Remember that the benefits of physical activity are to be enjoyed well beyond just your 28-day plan, and the best way to ensure that is the case is selecting movements you genuinely enjoy.

Cardio and Body Weight Exercises

Running: The quintessential and perhaps most well-recognized cardiovascular exercise.

Jumping jacks: Although 30 minutes straight of jumping jacks may be impractical, they are an excellent complement to the other activities on this list.

Dancing: Those who have a background in dancing may enjoy using it to their advantage, but anyone can put on their favorite songs and dance like there's nobody watching.

Jump rope: Own a jump rope? Why not use it as part of your cardiovascular workout? It is a fun way to get your cardio in.

Other options (equipment permitting): Activities like rowing, swimming and water aerobics, biking, and using elliptical and stair climbing machines can be great ways to exercise.

With the guidelines, your goal will be to work up to a total of 30 minutes of cardiovascular activity per workout session. You may use a combination of the exercises listed. I suggest that beginners should start with brisk walking or jogging—whatever activity you are most comfortable with.

Core

Plank: The plank is a classic core exercise that focuses on the stability and strength of the muscles in the abdominal and surrounding areas. Engage your buttocks, press your forearms into the ground, and hold for 60 seconds. Beginners may start with a 15- to 30-second hold and work their way up.

Side plank: Another core classic and a plank variation that focuses more on the oblique muscles on either side of your central abdominals. Keep the buttocks tight and prevent your torso from sagging to get the most out of this exercise.

Woodchopper: A slightly more dynamic movement that works the rotational functionality of your core and mimics chopping a log of wood. You can start with little to no weight until you feel comfortable and progress from there. Start the move with feet shoulder-width apart, back straight, and slightly crouched. If you are using weight, hold it with both hands next to the outside of either thigh, twist to the side, and lift the weight across and upward, keeping your arms straight and turning your torso such that you end up with the weight above your opposite shoulder.

Lower Body

Goblet squat: Start your stance with feet slightly wider than shoulder-width and a dumbbell held tightly with both hands in front of your chest. Sit back into a squat, hinging at both the knee and the hip joint, and lower your legs until they are parallel to the ground. Push up through your heels to the starting position and repeat. Use a chair to squat onto if you don't feel comfortable.

Dumbbell walking lunge: Start upright with a dumbbell in each hand and feet in your usual standing position. Step forward with one leg and sink until your back knee is just above the ground. Remain upright and ensure the front knee does not bend over the toes. Push through the heel of the front foot and step forward and through with your rear foot. Start with no weights and add weight as you feel comfortable.

Upper Body

Push-ups: These are the ultimate body-weight exercise and can be done just about anywhere. You will want to set up with your hands just beyond shoulder width, keeping your body in a straight line and always engaging your core as you ascend and descend, without letting your elbows flare out. Those who struggle to perform push-ups consecutively can start by performing them on their knees or even against a wall if regular push-ups sound like too much.

Dumbbell shoulder press: An excellent exercise for upper-body and shoulder strength. Bring a pair of dumbbells to ear level, palms forward, and straighten your arms overhead.

Full Body

Mountain climbers: On your hands and feet, keep your body in a straight line, with your abdominal and buttocks muscles engaged, similar to the top position of a push-up. Rapidly alternate pulling your knees into your chest while keeping your core tight. Continue in this left, right, left, right rhythm as if you are replicating a running motion. Always try to keep your spine in a straight line.

Push press: This is essentially a combination move incorporating a partial squat and a dumbbell shoulder press. Using a weight that you are comfortable with, stand feet slightly beyond shoulder width, with light dumbbells held in a pressing position. Descend for a squat to a depth you feel comfortable with, and on the ascent simultaneously push the dumbbells overhead.

Chapter 9: Additional Tips for Weight Loss

Understanding Habit

If you try to make a difference in your life, you're working to alter old habits and to create new ones. Sitting down and thinking about the improvements you want in your life is easy, but they are hard to execute and keep going. It's because you've produced patterns that need to be changed to be successful.

I have taught a lot of customers in my career, and almost every customer I teach knows what they have to do to achieve their target, but they can't. How do you do that?

Since they don't choose to take the necessary action periodically to develop habits that will produce long-term results.

Our customs control our actions. Understanding habits and their role in your life is essential, as they are responsible for your daytime choices. An individual does not lose weight because he or she is not aware that during commercial breaks, he or she is used to going to the kitchen to eat. For some instances, habit is something we don't know about. We do so consciously. Being mindful of your habits gives you the strength to make your life-changing decision. It's hard to make a decision when you know what your options are.

It's essential to be mindful of your old habits and the new ones you need to create while you are making changes in your life. Just think about the change you'd like to make. (Lose weight, get in shape, and get more energy) Now think about where you are right now, and what shift you want to make. (Lose 30 lbs., have more stamina, build strength, have more energy) Now think about the past and the acts you've taken, which are responsible for where you're at. (Eat fast food, watch TV, and drink too much every night).

Now ask yourself what actions do I need to take to bring about the change that I want to see in my life? The solutions you'll come up with are the acts you need to turn into behaviors. A habit is something you do, and you do not worry about it. You need to do the behavior regularly to build this habit before you have to think about it.

Habits aren't instantly created. It's something you have to do, consistently, for an extended period. How long does it take to do this? When you do it, and you do not have to worry about it. I read a lot of different stuff about how long it takes to build a habit ... Thirty days, sixty, ninety days ... I think these are fantastic goals, but I know it may take you a little longer. If this is a move that you want to make, you're going to do the research and work hard to make it happen.

Habits can be divided into two categories: motor and (actually) mental habits.

We reflect daily ways of acting or thinking we know without grappling with our will or even voluntary strength. Habits are acquired by learning, and then particularly by repetition.

It is, therefore, essential that the components (acts or thoughts) be replicated regularly and several times until a new habit is created.

Running, walking, walking, driving and so on are things that we had to know.

When we understand habits, we usually think of the behavior we replicate, and the habit of science will tell us why we replicate our patterns and develop habits as we grow up.

Habits are also repeated patterns of actions and behaviors that we are conditioned to perform, and that can evolve over many years, and habits that have evolved over many years are more likely to be stronger than those that have been developed recently or in a few years.

And habits that we learn as children remain with us all our lives are more likely than habits that we learn as adults. And the frequency or success of those habits would be directly linked to how long we have had those patterns of behavior.

And this is the routine that we all formed as children waking up in the morning and brushing our teeth. Now we have to wonder what if we're trying to stop the habits? What if we wake up and have not brushed our teeth? Besides the fact that we can end up with bad breath when we don't obey one of our everyday routines, there are real psychological effects of physical and emotional or social distress!

Brushing your teeth is a case in point. Another could be when you enter your apartment and turn on the TV or computer shortly after you return home. In your immediate area, you immediately feel uncomfortable if you stop doing so, even if it's your own home, as though something is missing from your life.

Suppose your TV or laptop is broken down, you can't exercise the habit, and you feel depressed. We, humans, are slaves to these patterns of behavior, and thus habits are an important part of our lives. This discomfort we feel can be seen as the product of 'habit obstruction' when we are unable to exercise our habits. Thus, the effects of disruption of habit may have a significant effect on our emotional, social and personal lives.

If habit obstruction effect is long-term, that is when your laptop is broken for weeks or months. You can't turn it on when you enter your house or apartment, and the habit obstruction effect will spread to habit hunger. After a few weeks of habit obstruction, you may even start losing your habit subconsciously when you get into the habit hunger effect.

So, habit hunger can cause some form of amnesia from your usual behavior, and you forget about that habit. It's all very good, but then not so simple, because you might have some form of habit displacement in this case and develop some other habit.

The Importance of Habits

Behind every habit, there is a real need that you need to satisfy. Be it any kind of habit, good or bad. Like for example:

· Who smokes to relieve stress?

· Who drinks to relax?

· Whoever exercises for pleasure?

All of these activities, whether harmful or not, contain a yearning for fulfilment for those who practice. This is what makes a habit so challenging to change.

So much so that when trying to change a habit, you will experience great difficulty in the first few weeks.

Because, when you stop doing something that was already customary, your body will begin to crave that sensation caused by that old custom that you left behind.

Tips to improve your habits

Life is full of habits, good and bad, it is just as easy to have positive habits as negative, but transforming them implies an effort and a lot of willpower, a change of beliefs and appreciation. The answer is in you, can you change your habits?

· Know the habits you would like to adopt. Start by making a detailed list of the habits you would like to change or improve.

· Analyze the attitudes that general conflicts. If you have not been able to identify all the bad habits or do not think you do not have them, ask yourself what kind of behaviors generate conflicts in your daily life and with the people around you, an example would be if you arrive at your appointments late and this causes discomfort in other people if you have no energy because you do not eat healthily or if you are a little overweight and you dislike it.

· Become aware of the importance of changing bad habits. It is important to raise awareness subtly to the people closest to you about the importance of improving their habits. If they do it simultaneously, it will be easier to adopt them. For example, if someone in your family buys junk food and you are looking for a healthy diet, it is vital to encourage them not to do so that everyone improves their habits and their diet, especially if this person is overweight.

· Build an action plan. Once you have identified the habits you would like to adopt, you need to make an action plan to carry it out. The first step is to become aware of the habit you want to change and continuously monitor your actions and thinking patterns to identify why you react that way. The next thing will be to repeat the new habit every day for at least 30 days, and it is the minimum time in which a habit is adopted. For example, if you want to start exercising, do it at least four days a week for two months. In this way, your body and mind will adapt to the new activities you do.

· Be honest with yourself. Finally, you must be objective and recognize if you have continued repeating the new habits, analyze if you already feel that they are part of your daily life. If not, it is important to examine the causes that prevented you from achieving it.

Habits are nothing more than the daily repetition of an attitude and discipline. The best day to start changing your habits is today. If you stop to think about all the time it takes to change a habit, and you probably won't, the important thing is to be determined and start today.

How to Improve Your Eating Habits for Weight Loss

The barriers people have reached for themselves seem to have no end in sight. Hunger, fruit diets and uncooked foods are among the drastic alternatives to the long old weight-loss problem. I had attempted to try these for myself, and none of them succeeded until I closed the diet and only changed my weight loss eating habits.

The diets are similar to weight loss band-aids. In a short-term illness, they are a fast solution and do not change behavior, metabolism or produce a true bang on body fat. Dietary rigidity does not increase the element of success; in reality, it decreases it. It is much easier to make gradual changes that are not upsetting or penalizing but launch the body on the road to equilibrium and its normal set point to some extent. Stable changes in eating habits are certainly an excellent option for losing weight.

Rather than eliminating calories by the end of the day or for a big meal, five or six small food portions are much healthier for the body. This sounds contradictory but real. The body burns calories in everyday exercise. This requires food calories to feed and digest. Reports show that up to 10% of calories are used to process the food.

Therefore, 50 calories are needed for food processing for a 500-calorie serving. It's been shown that eating less often helps in weight gain over the long term. To strengthen your weight-loss eating habits, you will regularly consume yet healthy foods. A psychosomatic eating benefit is feeling good. The feeling you're not hollow is beneficial in continuing the weight loss cycle.

Booming weight loss isn't a major science, nor does it entail difficulty and pain—easy changes like cooking nutritious meals 5-6 times a day. Eating the right part size is critical. Eating the right calories is important, and daily exercise is important. Eat and consume the right form of food are the safest dietary habits for weight loss.

Chapter 10: Love Your Body and Your Soul

Glad individuals acknowledge and love themselves regardless of what their body resembles, irrespective of how they feel. An ideal organization isn't preferred or all the more empowering over a body not considered immaculate by the "powers that be." Your magnificence originates from inside.

Consider somebody you know (or knew) who isn't generally all that appealing; however, who appears to adore herself so much that she feels delightful and acts as needs be. Individuals like that tend to be well known. Curiously, their excellence sparkles so splendidly that they seem, by all accounts, to be alluring to others.

Individuals in the media don't typically seem as though they seem to look in front of an audience or magazines and films. That is the reason the calling of make-up specialists exists. In my mind, what they do is make-up how this individual will appear to the crowd and fans. When photograph distributing is included, nobody is viewed as they look. All pictures get finished up.

At the point when you love yourself, honestly and genuinely love yourself, regardless of how old you develop to be your sentiments about you won't change. The fascinating piece about adoring yourself is living in a condition of satisfaction. Hardly any individuals get the chance to abide there—the individuals who do remain youthful until the end of time.

Tips to Assist You with Adoring Your Body

1. Take power back to characterize your Beauty

You are not just taking it back for the social/media definitions yet in addition to individuals around you in your life who have offered critical comments about your body. These individuals couldn't see the magnificence of your body since they had retained the standard definitions themselves and were deciding for you and most likely their body against these gauges too. Pause for a minute presently to close your eyes and envision reclaiming the power to characterize the excellence of your body. Take it once again from the social definitions and the media in your mental state, "I won't permit you to characterize what my body ought to resemble any longer." Think back to individuals that had offered

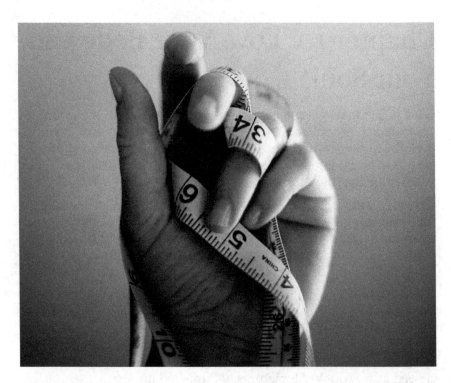

negative remarks to you about your body a relative, a sentimental accomplice, or different children when you were close to nothing. State to them in your mind, "I reclaim the power to characterize the magnificence of my body your remarks were bends and false, and I no longer give them any power." Feel how great this feels to free yourself from the entirety of this cynicism.

2. Clear Your Negative Beliefs about Your Body

Due to your introduction to the social molding about the alleged perfect female body you presumably have rehearsed self-judgment of your body for not fitting in with the advanced "perfect." These decisions and negative convictions are again contortions and not founded on the reality of the one of your very kind stunner body. We, as a whole, have groups of various sizes and shapes that are uncommon and genuinely delightful.

Relinquish your unbending convictions about how your body should look and start to perceive how the very things that are diverse about your body are the very things that make you one of a kind and lovely. Record the negative messages that you state to yourself about your body. Envision thinking of them to discharge them from your cognizance. Get them hard and fast, the most negative terrible ones you can consider. Take a gander at these messages, notice how you could never fantasy about directing these sentiments toward any other person in your life. Take a gander at all of these messages and apologize to your body, saying, "I'm sorry to such an extent that I directed these harmful sentiments toward you, I guarantee that I won't direct these sentiments toward you again and I will begin adoring you." Look at these messages again and with an expectation to completely discharge them destroy the piece of paper and discard it. A few people like to fabricate a fire outside and consume the document as a method of releasing this cynicism.

3. Exercise for the Joy of Feeling Your Body Move

At the point when you exercise to take out fat from your body as well as to make up for calories, eaten this can emerge out of a position of fear and have a vitality of attempting to control and battle against your body. Envision practicing for the delight of moving your body and from a goal to be wanting to your body, a craving for it to be sound and have more vitality. The customers I work with around this issue will, in general, have the option to keep up an activity program if they do it from a position of satisfaction and self-love as opposed to control and fear about their weight.

Notice if there are things throughout your life that you don't accomplish for fear of individuals seeing your body, like swimming, moving, or any other movement. Remind yourself that you have the right to do the things you appreciate regardless of your shape. Relinquish what others consider you and remain concentrated on the way that you reserve each option to do the things you understand.

4. Remind Yourself What the Purpose of Having a Body Is

Your body is yours to encounter life; ultimately, to take it in and appreciate it. Your body is a vehicle for you to encounter existence with the entirety of your faculties. Your body permits you: to feel a warm breeze on your skin, feel the cold water in a lake when you swim, see the entirety of the striking shades of nightfall, hear the whole of the excellence of the music, to listen to the hints of fowls and trees moving in the breeze, feel the non-abrasiveness of somebody's hand, feel the delight of moving, taste and appreciate flavorful food, communicate through a grin, tears or giggling.

Your body is for you, for nobody else to investigate or pass judgment. You are not here as a presentation for other people; however, as a wholly encapsulated person with more profound, more extravagant characteristics than merely your appearance.

5. at the point when you look in The Mirror-Look at Yourself through Loving Eyes

For some, ladies glancing in the mirror transforms into an activity of self-judgment. They focus on the entirety of their apparent flaws and what they feel is "off-base" with their body or face. Again, the models they are deciding for themselves against is this ridiculous perfect that is advanced in the media. I have numerous customers who, when they previously began working with me, said that they couldn't glance in the mirror since all they saw were these apparent flaws. I recommend that they move this by instead taking a gander at themselves in the mirror through adoring eyes. A model would be if you look in the mirror and see a wrinkle that you would generally judge, see this wrinkle with affection and empathy and even observe the excellence of this wrinkle. Set an away from to see yourself through the perspective of adoration intrude on the self-judgment and move into being exceptionally cherishing with yourself. This will be something that you have to rehearse before it turns into a propensity. Yet, it will be justified even despite the exertion since you will start to feel extremely magnificent about yourself.

6. Have Your Self-Esteem be Internally Referenced

Have your self-regard be founded on your interior characteristics as opposed to your outside appearance. What are the features that make yourself you? Is it your sympathy, your new innovativeness, your insight, your ability to have a ton of fun, your awareness, your perceptiveness, your ability to tune in to individuals, or your caring heart? Think about the individuals that you love in your life. You love them for what their identity is, the one of a kind Spirit that they are, not for what they resemble. That is how they feel about you, they love you for what your identity is and the entirety of the extraordinary characteristics that make up you. Figure out how to esteem yourself for the substance of you, not for the physical structure that you travel around in.

7. Investigate the deeper purpose behind the distraction with your appearance/weight.

Here and there, when somebody is engrossed with their

appearance, it might be a shirking system for more profound, increasingly agonizing sentiments. Check-in with yourself and check whether this may be the situation. If in your youth things were excruciating for you and crazy, you may have figured out how to concentrate on your weight as an approach to keep away from the forlornness and defenselessness of what was going on around you. Or then again, perhaps there is a problematic issue in your life today that you don't have the fearlessness to confront like a problematic relationship or absence of direction in your life. A distraction with your appearance occupies you from facing these issues. If so, for you, it is significant for you to get support for yourself to open up to confront these sentiments straightforwardly. You can get this help through facing the challenge to uncover your feelings to a confided in companion or working with an advocate who can assist you with working through these emotions.

8. Take out Comparing Yourself to Others

The vitality of correlation and rivalry is damaging to yourself and the other individual. Doing this is simply one more type of putting yourself and won't help you to feel better; however, it will exacerbate you think even. Pledge to pass on this sort of vitality. Instead, if you see somebody who is appealing as opposed to contrasting yourself with this individual or making a decision about them, the state instead, "She is alluring as am I." Celebrate that other individual and yourself as well. You will discover this feels such a significant amount of superior to contrasting yourself with them or being basic.

9. Take One of the Areas of Your Body You Typically Judge and Take a Week to Fully Love This Part of You

Go through 15 minutes daily taking a gander at this piece of your body, and discover things to adore about it, even better, do it for the day. The additionally testing it is to do this, the more you have to do it! I read in a book about a lady who did this activity, and following seven days of doing it, an outsider came up to her and revealed to her how delightful this piece of her body was! At the point when we change our particular manner of seeing ourselves, it changes the style in which others see us as well. You need your first expectation of doing this activity to be simply the move in your affection, not to have an impact on how others see you. How you see you are continually going to be what is generally significant.

Chapter 11: Lose Weight Fast and Naturally

Numerous individuals are uncertain about how to lose weight securely and normally. It does not support that multiple sites and notices, especially those having a place with companies that sell diet drugs or other weight-loss products, promote misinformation about losing weight.

As indicated by 2014 research, a great many people who look for tips on the most proficient method to get thinner will go over false or deluding information on weight reduction.

"Fad" diets and exercise regimens can at times be hazardous as they can keep individuals from meeting their nourishing needs.

As indicated by the Centers for Disease Control and Prevention, the most secure measure of weight to lose every week is somewhere in the range of 1 and 2 pounds. The individuals who suffer substantially more every week or attempt craze diets or projects are significantly more prone to recover weight.

1. **Keeping Refreshing Bites at Home and In the Workplace**

Individuals frequently pick to eat nourishments that are helpful, so it is ideal to abstain from keeping prepackaged tidbits and confections close by.

One investigation found that individuals who kept unhealthful nourishment at home thought that it was increasingly hard to keep up or lose weight.

Keeping healthful snacks at home and work can enable an individual to meet their nourishing needs and maintain a strategic distance from an abundance of sugar and salt. Great snack choices include:

- nuts with no added salt or sugar
- natural products
- prechopped vegetables
- low-fat yoghurts
- dried seaweed

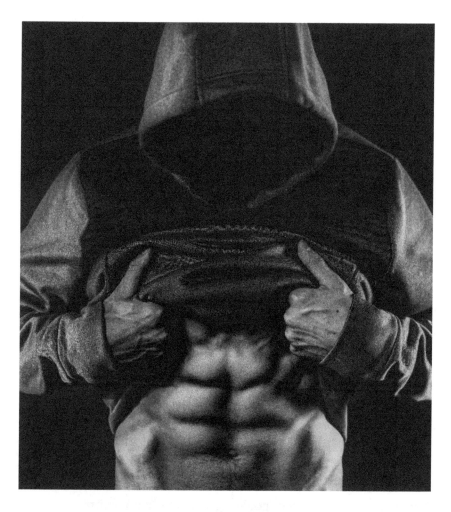

2. Removing Processed Foods

Processed foods are high in sodium, fat, calories, and sugar. They frequently contain fewer supplements than entire nourishments.

As indicated by a primer research study, processed foods are substantially more likely than different food sources to prompt addictive eating practices, which will, in general, outcome in individuals indulging.

3. Eating More Protein

An eating routine high in protein can enable an individual to lose weight. A diagram of existing examination on high protein eats fewer carbs inferred that they are an effective system for forestalling or treating obesity.

The information demonstrated that higher-protein diets of 25–30 grams of protein for each feast gave enhancements in hunger, bodyweight the board, cardiometabolic hazard components, or these wellbeing results.

- fish
- beans, peas, and lentils
- white poultry
- low-fat cottage cheese
- tofu

4. Stopping Included Sugar

Sugar is not in every case simple to maintain a strategic distance from; however, disposing of handled nourishments is a positive initial step to take.

As per the National Cancer Institute, men matured 19 years and more established devour a normal of more than 19 teaspoons of included sugar a day. Ladies in a similar age bunch eat more than 14 teaspoons of added sugar a day.

A significant part of the sugar that individuals devour originates from fructose, which the liver separates and transforms into fat. After the liver converts the sugar into fat, it discharges these fat cells into the blood, which can prompt weight gain.

5. Drinking Black Coffee

Coffee may have some constructive wellbeing impacts if an individual forgoes, including sugar and fat. The writers of a survey article saw that coffee improved the body's processing of carbohydrates and fats.

A like look at featured a relationship between coffee utilization and a lower danger of diabetes and liver disease.

6. Remaining Hydrated

Water is the best liquid that an individual can drink for the day. It contains no calories and gives an abundance of health benefits.

At the point when an individual drinks water for the day, the water helps increment their digestion. Drinking water before a feast can likewise help decrease the sum that they eat.

At long last, if individuals supplant sweet refreshments with water, this will help decrease all outnumber of calories that they devour for the day.

7. Keeping Away from The Calories in Beverages

Soft drinks, natural product squeezes, and sports and caffeinated drinks regularly contain abundant sugar, which can prompt weight increase and make it progressively hard for an individual to get in shape.

Other high-calorie drinks incorporate liquor and strength espressos, like lattes, which contain milk and sugar.

Individuals can have a go at supplanting, at any rate, one of these drinks every day with water, shining water with lemon, or an herbal tea.

8. Avoiding Refined Carbohydrates

Proof in The American Journal of Clinical Nutrition recommends that refined sugars might be more harmful to the body's digestion than saturated fats.

Considering the convergence of sugar from refined starches, the liver will make and discharge fat into the circulatory system.

To diminish weight and keep it off, an individual can eat entire grains.

Refined or simple carbohydrates incorporate the accompanying nourishments:

- white rice
- white bread
- white flour
- candies
- numerous sorts of cereal
- included sugars
- numerous sorts of pasta

Rice, bread, and pasta are, for the most part, accessible in entire grain varieties, which can help weight reduction and help shield the body from disease.

9. Fasting in Cycles

Fasting for short periods may enable an individual to get more fit.

As per a recent report, irregular fasting or substitute day fasting can allow an individual to get in shape and keep up their weight reduction.

However, not every person should quick. Fasting can be dangerous for kids, creating adolescents, pregnant ladies, older individuals, and individuals with hidden wellbeing conditions.

10. Counting Calories and Keeping A Nourishment Diary

Counting calories can be a viable method to abstain from gorging. By tallying calories, an individual will know about precisely the amount they are devouring. This mindfulness can assist them with removing superfluous calories and settle on better dietary decisions.

A nourishment diary can enable an individual to consider what and the amount they are devouring each day. By doing this, they can likewise guarantee that they are getting enough of each stimulating nutrition type, for example, vegetables and proteins.

11. Brushing Teeth Between Dinners or Prior at Night

Notwithstanding improving dental cleanliness, brushing the teeth can help lessen the impulse to nibble between dinners.

If an individual who regularly snacks around evening time brushes their teeth prior at night, they may feel less enticed to eat extra snacks.

12. Eating More Fruits and Vegetables

An eating routine wealthy in products of the soil can enable an individual to get more fit and keep up their weight reduction.

The author of an orderly survey supports this case, expressing that advancing an expansion in products of the soil utilization is probably not going to cause any weight increase, even without instructing individuals to diminish their use regarding different nourishments.

13. Lessening Carbohydrate Consumption

Diets low in basic starches can enable an individual to reduce their weight by constraining the measure of added sugar that they eat.

Restorative low carbohydrate abstains from food center around expending entire sugars, high fats, fiber, and lean proteins. Rather than restricting all sugars for a brief period, this ought to be a reasonable, long haul dietary alteration.

14. Eating More Fiber

Fiber offers a few potential advantages to an individual hoping to get thinner. Research in Nutrition expresses that an expansion in fiber utilization can enable an individual to feel fuller more rapidly.

Furthermore, fiber helps weight reduction by advancing absorption and adjusting the microorganisms in the gut.

15. Expanding Traditional Cardiovascular and Resistance Training

Numerous individuals do not practice regularly and may likewise have inactive occupations. It is critical to incorporate both cardiovascular (cardio) work out, for example, running or strolling, and opposition preparing in a regular exercise program.

Cardio enables the body to consume calories rapidly while obstruction preparing manufactures fit bulk. Bulk can assist individuals with consuming more calories very still.

Furthermore, explore has discovered that individuals who take an interest in high-intensity interval training (HIIT) can lose more weight and see more prominent enhancements in their cardiovascular wellbeing than individuals who are utilizing other mainstream strategies for weight reduction.

16. Devouring Whey Protein

Individuals who use whey protein may expand their slender bulk while diminishing muscle versus fat, which can help with weight reduction.

Research from 2014 found that whey protein, in the mix with practice or a weight reduction diet, may help diminish body weight and muscle to fat ratio.

17. Eating Slowly

Eating slowly can enable an individual to decrease all outnumber of calories that they expend in one sitting. The purpose behind this is it can require some investment to understand that the stomach is full.

One examination showed that eating rapidly relates to corpulence. While the investigation couldn't prescribe mediations to enable an individual to eat all the more gradually, the outcomes do propose that eating nourishment at a slower pace can help decrease calorie consumption.

Biting nourishment completely and eating at a table with others may enable an individual to back off while eating.

18. Including Chili

Adding spice to nourishments may enable an individual to get more fit. Capsaicin is a compound that is normally present in flavors, for example, bean stew powder, and may have constructive outcomes.

For instance, inquire about demonstrates that capsaicin can assist ignite with fatting and increment digestion, yet at low rates.

19. Getting More Sleep

There is a link between corpulence and an absence of value rest. The research proposes that getting adequate rest can add to weight loss. The researchers found that ladies who depicted their rest quality as poor or reasonable were more averse to effectively get in shape than the individuals who detailed their rest quality as being generally excellent.

20. Utilizing a Smaller Plate

Utilizing smaller plates could have a positive mental impact. Individuals will, in general, fill their plate, so lessening the size of the plate may help decrease the measure of nourishment that an individual eats in one sitting. A 2015 systematic reassessment inferred that diminishing plate size could affect partition control and vitality utilization, yet it was hazy whether this was material over the full scope of bit sizes. Individuals hoping to get in shape securely and normally should concentrate on making a perpetual way of life changes instead of embracing brief measures.

Individuals must concentrate on making changes that they can keep up. Now and again, an individual may want to execute changes steadily or take a stab at presenting each in turn.

Any individual who thinks that it is difficult to get more fit may profit by addressing a specialist or dietitian to discover an arrangement that works for them.

Chapter 12: Changing Your Mindset

Why a Rigid and Aggressive Approach Doesn't Work

When it comes to making any sort of change in life, the approach you take will make or break your success. If you choose a strategy that doesn't work well with your specific personality, the likelihood of relapse occurring will be extremely high. We will discuss the drawbacks of approaching change with an aggressive and rigid approach.

Taking an approach that is focused on perfection leaves you feeling down on yourself and like a failure most of the time. Because this causes you to notice that you are not perfect instead of focusing on the right parts, the progress you have made will always make you feel like you are not doing enough or that you have not made enough progress. Since you will never achieve perfection as this is impossible for anyone, you will never feel satisfaction or allow yourself to celebrate your achievements. You must recognize that this will be something complicated, but that you will do it anyways. If you force yourself into change like a drill sergeant and with an aggressive mindset, you will end up beating yourself up every day for something. Pushing yourself will not lead to a long-lasting change, as you will eventually become fed up with all the rules you have placed on yourself, and you will just want to abandon the entire mission. If you approach the change with rigidity, you will not allow yourself time to look back on your achievements and celebrate yourself, to have a tasty meal that is good for your soul every once in a while, and you may fall off of your plan in a more extreme way than you were before. You may end up having a week-long binge and dropping down into worse habits than you had back.

Your mindset plays a huge role in your success when it comes to change. The way that you view your journey will make or break it and will determine whether or not your change is lasting or fleeting, and whether or not you become invested in making the changes in your life. While you need to push yourself to do anything hard, the key is knowing when to ease up on yourself a little bit and when to push harder. Recognizing and responding to this is much more useful than putting your nose to the grindstone

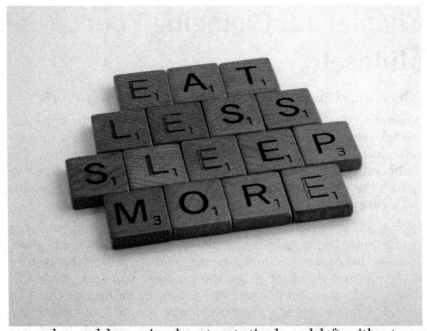

every day and becoming burnt out, tired, and left without any more willpower. Continuing on this challenging journey that a lifestyle change involves, you must give yourself a break now and then. Think of this like running a marathon where you will need to go about it slowly and purposefully with a strategy in mind. If you ran into a marathon full-speed and refused to slow down or look back at all, you would lose energy, stamina, and motivation in quite a short amount of time and turn back or run off the side of the road feeling defeated and as if you failed. Looking at this example, you can see that this person did not fail. They just approached the marathon with the wrong strategy and that they would have been completely capable of finishing that marathon if they had taken their time, followed a plan, and slowed down every once in a while, to regain their strength. Even if they walked the marathon slowly for hours and hours, eventually, they would make it over that finish line. They would probably also do so feeling proud, accomplished, and like a new person. This is how we want to view this journey or any journey of self-improvement. Even if you take only one tiny step each day, you are making a step toward your goal, and that is the crucial part.

The Deprivation Trap

There is a term when it comes to dieting that is called The

Deprivation Trap. The deprivation trap is something that can occur when you approach dieting with a strict mindset. What this means is that you become stuck in a type of thinking trap within your mind. In this type of thinking, you become focused on what you can't have and what you are restricting yourself off. You become hyper-focused on everything you can't allow yourself to have and become resentful of the fact that you aren't able just to eat what you want. After a while, because you are focusing so intently on what you can't have and the fact that you can't have it, you decide that you are just going to have it anyway, or just have a little bit of it, out of a feeling of anger and entitlement. The next thing you know, you have gone on a binge, and after restricting yourself entirely for some time, you have now undone that in a single sitting. You will then begin to feel terrible about yourself and what you have done, and you begin to feel like you need to punish yourself. Thus can start the cycle of deprivation.

Further, it is quite challenging to avoid this when you are trying to make a change by using deprivation. It is quite rare that a person, no matter how strong their willpower, will be able to deprive themselves of something without easing off of it ultimately. A sudden and strict deprivation is not natural to our brains and will leave us feeling confused and frustrated.

How to Overcome the Deprivation Trap

To avoid the deprivation trap or overcome it if you are already finding yourself there, there are things that we can do and approaches we can take that will set us up better for success.

To avoid this trap, the first thing we must do is prevent complete deprivation of anything. Instead of depriving ourselves of something ultimately, we will instead try to make better choices, one meal or one snack at a time. Focusing on small parts of our day or lower sections of our lives will help us to motivate ourselves. This is because looking forward to the rest of our lives and thinking that we will never be able to have a sure thing again is quite an overwhelming thought, especially if this is something that we enjoy. Therefore, we must instead look at it like "I will make a better choice for my lunch today," and then all you need to focus on is lunch, not the entire rest of your life.

Strategies for the Mind

Like we all know and read in some websites about weight-loss, easing into a lifestyle change is the best way to go about something like this because of the way that our minds work. We don't like looking forward to our lives and feeling like we will have no control over what we are going to do with it. By choosing smaller sections to break it up into, we can be more present in each moment, which makes making healthy choices easier. By doing so, all of these small sections add up to weeks, months, and eventually years of healthy options. Finally, we have gone a year without turning to sweets in a moment of sadness and only chosen them when we are consciously choosing to treat ourselves.

Another strategy that we can use for our minds is to reward yourself at milestones along your journey. At one week you can reward yourself with a date night at a restaurant, or at one month you can visit the new bakery down the street. This not only helps you to stay motivated because you are allowing yourself some of the joys you love, but it also keeps you motivated because you are allowing yourself to take time to look back at how far you have come and feel great about your progress. Allowing yourself to celebrate goes hand in hand with this, as well. When you make the right choice or plan what you will order at a restaurant before you get there, allowing yourself to feel happy and proud is very important. By doing this, you are showing yourself that you have done something great, that you are capable of making changes, and that you will allow yourself to feel good about these positive strides you have made instead of just looking to the next one all the time. If you were to ignore this and be of the mindset that nothing is good enough, you would end up feeling burnt out and entirely down about the length of the process. Think of that marathon analogy again, and this is what can happen if we don't allow ourselves time to feel proud and accomplished for small victories along the way.

Another strategy for the mind is to avoid beating yourself up for falling off the wagon. This may happen sometimes. What we need to do, though, is to focus not on the fact that it has happened, but on how we are going to deal with and react to it. There are a variety of reactions that a person can have to this. We will examine the possible responses and the pros and cons below:

One is that they feel as though their progress is ruined and that they might as well begin another time again, so they go back to their old ways and may not try again for some time. This could happen many times over as they will fall off each time and then decide that they might as well give up this time and try again, but each time it ends the same.

Two, the person could fall off of their diet plan and tell themselves that this day is a write-off and that they will begin the next day again. The problem with this method is that continuing the rest of the day as you would have before you decided to make a change will make it so that the next day is like beginning all over again, and it will be tough to start again. They may be able to start the next day again, and it could be fine, but they must be able to motivate themselves if they are to do this. Knowing that you have fallen off makes it so that you may feel down on yourself and feel as though you can't do it, so beginning again the next day is significant.

And they then decide that they will pick it up again the next week. This will be even harder than starting the next day again as multiple days of eating whatever you like will make it very hard to go back to making the healthy choices still afterwards.

Four, after eating something that they wish they hadn't, and that wasn't a healthy choice, they will decide not to eat anything for the rest of the day so that they don't eat too many calories or too much sugar, and decide that the next day they will begin again. This is very difficult on the body as you are going to be quite hungry by the time bed rolls around. Instead of forgiving yourself, you are punishing yourself, and it will make it very hard not to reach for chips late at night when you are starving and feeling down.

Chapter 13: Why Is It Hard to Lose Weight?

For anyone who has ever struggled with weight, life can seem like an uphill battle. It can be downright devastating to see how difficult it can be to turn things around and shed some weight.

The fact of the matter is that losing weight doesn't have to be an uphill battle. Most of this requires you to understand better why this struggle happens and what you can do to help give yourself a fighting chance.

Physiological factors are affecting your ability to lose weight. There are also psychological, emotional and even spiritual causes that affect your overall body's ability to help you lose weight and reach your ideal weight levels.

The Obvious Culprits

The obvious culprits that are holding you back are diet, a lack of exercise and a combination of both.

First off, your diet plays a crucial role in your overall health and wellbeing. When it comes to weight management, your diet has everything to do with your ability to stay in shape and ward of unwanted weight.

When it comes to diet, we are not talking about keto, vegan, or Atkins; we are talking about the common foods which you consume and the amounts that you have of each one which is why diet is one of the obvious culprits. If you have a diet that is high in fat, high in sodium and high in sugar, you can rest assured that your body will end up gaining weight at a rapid rate.

When you consume high amounts of sugar, carbs and fats, your body transforms them into glucose which storing it in the body as fat. Of course, a proportion of the glucose produced by your body is used up as energy. However, if you consume far more than you need, your body isn't going to get rid of it; your body is going to hold on to it and make sure that it is stored for a rainy day.

Here is another vital aspect to consider: sweet and salty foods, the kind that we love so dearly, trigger "happy hormones" in the brain, namely dopamine. Dopamine is a hormone that is released by the body when it "feels good". And the food is one of the best

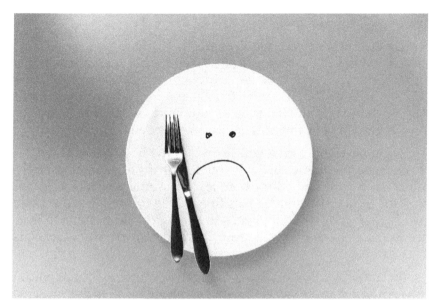

ways to trigger it, which is why you somehow feel better after eating your favorite meals. It also explains the reason why we resort to food when we are not feeling well, which is called "comfort food", and it is one of the most popular coping mechanisms employed by folks around the world.

This rush of dopamine causes a person to become addicted to food. As with any addiction, there comes a time when you need to get more and more of that same substance to meet your body's requirements.

As a result of diet, a lack of regular exercise can do a number on your ability to lose weight and maintain a healthy balance. What regular exercise does is increase your body's overall caloric requirement. As such, your metabolism needs to convert fat at higher rates to keep up with your body's energy demands.

As the body's energetic requirements increase, that is, as your exercise regimen gets more and more intense, you will find that you will need increased amounts of both oxygen and glucose which is one of the reasons why you feel hungrier when you ramp up your workouts.

However, increased caloric intake isn't just about consuming more and more calories for the sake of consuming more and more calories; you need to consume an equal amount of proteins, carbs, fats and vitamins too for your body to build the necessary elements that will build muscle, foster movement and provide proper oxygenation in the blood.

Moreover, nutrients are required for the body to recover. One of the byproducts of exercise is called "lactic acid". Lactic acid builds up in the muscles as they get more and more tired. Lactic acid signals the body that it is time to stop working out or risk injury if you continue. Without lactic acid, your body would have no way of knowing when your muscles have overextended their capacity.

After you have completed your workout, the body needs to get rid of the lactic acid buildup. So, if you don't have enough of the right minerals in your body, for example, potassium, your muscles will ache for days until your body is finally able to get rid of the lactic acid buildup. This example goes to show how proper nutrition is needed to help the body get moving and also recover once it is done exercising.

As a result, a lack of exercise reconfigures your body's metabolism to work at a slower pace. What that means is that you need to consume fewer calories to fuel your body's lack of exercise. So, if you end up wasting more than you need, your body will just put it away for a rainy day. Plain and simple.

The Sneaky Culprits

The sneaky culprits are the ones that aren't quite so overt in causing you to gain weight or have trouble shedding pounds. These culprits hide beneath the surface but are very useful when it comes to keeping you overweight. The first culprit we are going to be looking at is called "stress".

Stress is a potent force. From an evolutionary perspective, it exists as a means of fueling the flight-or-fight response. Stress is the human response to danger. When a person senses danger, the body begins to secrete a hormone called "cortisol". When cortisol begins running through the body, it signals the entire system to prep for a potential showdown. Depending on the situation, it might be best to hightail it out and live to fight another day.

In our modern way of life, stress isn't so much a response to life and death situations (though it can certainly be). Instead, it is the response to cases that are deemed as "conflictive" by the mind. This could be a confrontation with a co-worker, bumper to bumper traffic, or any other type of situation in which a person feels vulnerable in some way.

Throughout our lives, we subject to countless interactions in which we must deal with stress. In general terms, the feelings of alertness subside when the perceived threat is gone. However, when a person is exposed to prolonged periods of stress, any number of changes can happen.

One such change is overexposure to cortisol. When there is too much cortisol in the body, the body's overall response is to hoard calories, increase the production of other hormones such as adrenaline and kick up the immune system's function.

This response by the body is akin to the panic response that the body would assume when faced with prolonged periods of hunger or fasting. As a result, the body needs to go into survival mode. Please bear in mind that the body has no clue if it is being chased by a bear, dealing with a natural disaster or just having a bad day at the office. Regardless of the circumstances, the body is faced with the need to ensure its survival. So, anything that it eats goes straight to fat stores.

Moreover, a person's stressful situation makes them search for comfort and solace. There are various means of achieving this. Food is one of them. So is alcohol consumption. These two types of pleasures lead to significant use of calories. Again, when the body is in high gear, it will store as many calories and keep them in reserve.

This what makes you gain weight when you are stressed out.

Another of the sneaky culprits is sleep deprivation. In short, sleep deprivation is sleeping less than the recommended 8 hours that all adults should sleep. In the case of children, the recommended amount of sleep can be anywhere from 8 to 12 hours, depending on their age.

Granted, some adults can function perfectly well with less than 8 hours' sleep. Some folks can work perfectly well with 6 hours' sleep while there are folks who are shattered when they don't get eight or even more hours' sleep. This is different for everyone as each individual is different in this regard.

That being said, sleep deprivation can trigger massive amounts of cortisol. This, fueled by ongoing exposure to stress, leads the body to further deepening its panic mode. When this occurs, you can rest assured that striking a healthy balance between emotional wellbeing and physical health can be nearly impossible to achieve.

Now, the best way to overcome sleep deprivation is to get sleep.

But that is easier said than done. One of the best ways to get back on track to a certain degree is to get in enough sleep when you can.

The last sneaky culprit on our list is emotional distress. Emotional distress can occur as a result of any number of factors. For example, the loss of a loved one, a stressful move, a divorce, or the loss of a job can all contribute to large amounts of emotional distress. While all the situations mentioned above begin as a stressful situation, they can fester and lead to severe psychological issues. Over time, these emotional issues can grow into more profound topics such as General Anxiety Disorder or Depression. Studies have shown that prolonged periods of stress can lead to depression and a condition known as Major Depression.

The most common course of treatment for anxiety and depression is the use of an antidepressant. And guess what: one of the side effects associated with antidepressants is the weight. The reason for this is that antidepressant tinkers with the brain's chemistry in such a way that they alter the brain's processing of chemicals through the suppression of serotonin transport. This causes the brain to readjust its overall chemistry. Thus, you might find the body unable to process food quite the same way. In general, it is common to see folks gain as much as 10 pounds as a result of taking antidepressants.

As you can see, weight gain is not the result of "laziness" or being "undisciplined". Sure, you might have to clean up your diet somewhat and get more exercise. But the causes we have outlined here ought to provide you with enough material to see why there are less obvious causes that are keeping yours from achieving your ideal weight. This is why meditation plays such a key role in helping you deal with stress and emotional strife while helping you find a balance between your overall mental and physical wellbeing.

Ultimately, the strategies and techniques that we will further outline here will provide you with the tools that will help you strike that balance and eventually lead you to find the most effective way in which you will deal with the rigors of your day-to-day life while being able to make the most out of your efforts to lead a healthier life. You have everything you need to do it. So, let's find out how you can achieve this.

Chapter 14: Why You Should Stop Emotional Eating

We don't know we're an emotional eater for most of us, or we don't think it's that severe. For some of us, it doesn't lead to feelings of shame or weight gain. We can console some of us and think it's not a big deal, but it's not.

Among others, emotional eating is out of balance, something that can dominate our everyday lives. This may seem like overwhelming cravings or hunger, but it's just the feeling that we feel hungry, helpless and add to our weight.

Comfort food gives us immediate pleasure and takes away feeling. Digestion and sensation require a lot of time, and the body can't do it. Comfort eating helps us to suppress pain because we flood our digestive tract with poisonous waste.

When we feel anxious, feeling a big empty hole inside us like we're hungry can be natural. Instead of confronting what this means— i.e. our emotions—we're stuffing it down. In culture, it seems we are afraid to feel too much that we don't even know we're running from our feelings much of the time.

If we don't let ourselves react, we'll repress it. You will feel exhausted until you begin to let yourself feel the thoughts or feelings that emerge and avoid stuffing down. It is because the body releases past pent-up emotions, and it can strike you hard.

That's why it can be hard to let go of emotional eating, as we have to conquer the initial "scare" to move on and start learning to accept emotions for what they are. To be present, allowing a feeling to wash over us is wonderful and should be appreciated.

The more you allow yourself to be in the present moment and feel, the fewer feelings that overtake you, the less terrified you will be. The emotion's strength also decreases. You'll become mentally and physically stronger. When it's off your stomach, you'll feel so much better than replacing it with food.

Getting to this point isn't fast. Some people can split their emotional eating by better nourishing their bodies to get rid of

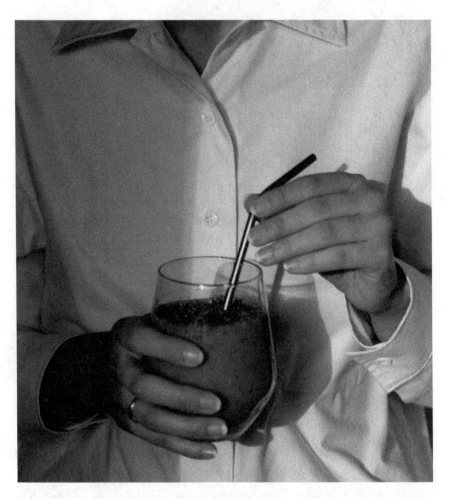

physical cravings and supporting others when they feel anxious or emotional.

To stop emotional eating, you must be mindful of how and why you eat—taking a day out to consider what makes you happy. Many people don't even understand real hunger!

When you're eating mentally, can you stop yourself?

Could you sit and let the emotion wash over you instead of eating, give yourself time to feel it and transfer it? Or would you talk to someone about how you feel?

Don't injure yourself.

Emotional eating is usually something you've done from an early age because it's part of your make-up. It's a practiced habit, so you've learned to cope with the environment.

It takes time to undo something so ingrained in you, so if you find yourself eating out of guilt, if you mess up, learn from it, just move on. Recognition is the first step. If you know you eat safely, you can conquer it.

Journaling will also help you recognize eating habits. Note down before, during and after a meal. What caused eating was real hunger?

To learn how to avoid emotional eating, I can help. For years, I suffered from an emotional eating epidemic, sometimes going on a day-to-day binge eating marathon. I never really understood what caused these eating outbursts, all I knew was that I would start eating and not stop until the food was gone, or anyone near me saw me.

The situation escalated, and my weight started to increase. Any diet I was on would instantly fail, and my self-confidence reached an all-time low. My eating causes were thought to be related to work stress, but so many others may play a part. Relationships, depression, financial difficulties, and many others will easily consume binge sequence.

When I started trying to figure out how to avoid emotional eating, I didn't know where to start. Like you, I went online and started investigating. I spent the whole day reading, digesting, and gathering emotional cure knowledge, then around 3 a.m. I found my savior that morning.

And how can you avoid emotional eating?

The answer is very easy. The trick is identifying the real root cause of the problems and addressing those root causes. You may think its tension or job issues. Yet mental eating disorders are also much more profound than on the surface. Following the root, a cause can quickly treat these symptoms and safely cure your binge eating.

Mental eating satisfies your mental appetite. It's not about your kitchen, but the issue lies in your head. What are the most powerful emotional eating challenge strategies?

List your food cravings to relax.

Distracting yourself doesn't mean being lazy in this situation. It's not like texting while driving, or you're out of control. When you hide from your food cravings, it means you're turning your focus to something else. It's more purposeful.

Do something or concentrate on another action or event. Whenever you feel like gorging food, try getting a piece of paper and list five items from five categories of something like the names of five people whenever you feel upset, angry or depressed.

Perhaps you should mention five ways to relax. If you want to calm down, what are your five places?

When anxious, what five feel-good phrases can you tell yourself? How about five things to stop eating?

Place on your fridge or kitchen cabinet after finishing this list. Next time you're overwhelmed by your persuasive food cravings, browse through your list and do one of the 25 things suggested there.

Prepare ahead for future emotional issues.

Over the weekend, grab a piece of paper and a pencil and take a path to your tasks in the days ahead. Your map reveals your expected exits and potential detours. Pick an emotionally consuming picture.

Place the icon over an event or activity that could cause your food cravings, like an early lunch with your in-laws. Prepare ahead for that case. Search for the restaurant menu online to order something delicious and nutritious.

Drop the concerns inside.

Whenever anxious, taking a deep breath helps. Another thing to detoxify yourself from stress is to do a visual trick. Breathe deeply and imagine a squeegee (that piece of cloth you use to clean your window or windshield) near your eyes. Slowly breathe out, picture the squeegee wiping clean inside. Delete all your concerns. Do it three times.

Self-talk like you're royalty. Self-criticism is usually emotional. Toxic words you say to yourself, such as "I'm such a loser" or "I can never seem to do anything right," force you to drive to the nearest. Don't be fooled by these claims, though brief.

Such feelings, like acid rain, slowly erode your well-being. The next time you're caught telling yourself these negative things, overcome by moving to a third-person perspective.

If you think "I'm such a mess," tell yourself then that "Janice is such a mess, but Janice will do what it takes to get things done and make herself happy."

This approach will get you out of the negative self-talk loop and have some perspective. Pull up and be positive and have the strength and avoid emotional eating.

Over-food is still not given enough consideration. It's always seen as not a serious problem to laugh at.

This is an incorrect view as a horrific condition needing urgent treatment. The positive thing is that you take action to help you avoid emotional eating forever. I know because I did it myself.

Step1-Recognize triggers

For each person, emotional eating is triggered differently. Some people get cravings when stressed out, some when depressed or bored. You need to try to work out the emotional causes. When you know what they are, you'll get an early notice when the urge to feed comes to you.

Step 2-Eliminate Temptation

One thing most people don't realize about emotional eating is that desire is always for one specific food. It's always ice-cream or candy for kids. It's still pizza for guys.

When you couldn't fulfil this lure, it won't bother you. Save your home from all of these temptations.

Throw out any nearby pizza delivery locations. Again, you know your tempters, so get rid of them and make overeating difficult.

Step 3-Break contact

It's instant and urgent when craving hits. You're fed RIGHT NOW! To stop this, you must break this immediate bond by taking sometime between desires and eating.

Call a friend Count to 60

Write down what you feel like

Do some exercises go out for a walk

Take a shower

What you can do to make the urge subside do wonder.

Take these three moves, and you'll soon take them better and conquer emotional eating for good.

Chapter 15: Hypnotic Gastric Band Techniques

If you would like to lose some weight without using surgery, then the hypnotic gastric band is the best tool for you. The hypnotic gastric band is the natural healthy eating tool that will help to control your appetite and your portion sizes. In this sense, hypnosis plays a significant role in helping you to lose weight without having to go through the risk that comes with surgery.

It is a subconscious suggestion that you already have, a gastric band comes intending to influence the body to respond by creating a feeling of satiety. It is now available in a public domain that dieting does not help to solve lifestyle challenges that are needed for weight loss and management.

Temporary diet plans are not effective while maintaining continuous plans are difficult. Notably, these plans are going to deprive you of your favorite foods, since they are too restrictive. Deep down within you, you might have a problem with your body's weight since diets have not worked for you in the past.

If you want to try something that will be able to provide a positive edge for you, then you should be able to control your cravings around food hypnotically. By reaching this point, you must try hypnosis, which has proven some results in aiding weight loss.

So now you can relax and take this time to wind yourself down and allow all those tensions to start flowing out and disappearing. So just bring to mind to remember that hypnosis is just self-hypnosis, that this is not something that someone will be able to do for you. Because hypnosis is simply a state of deep relaxation, which successfully helps you to bypass your critical factors so that the suggestions that are beneficial to your true self will be readily received and accepted by your deeper unconscious mind.

After all, trance is an everyday natural calming experience, and you are entering into that experience easily and effortlessly. So start by asking yourself, if you've ever put yourself in a calm relaxing state before this moment, and if so, you can recall all those calm and relaxing states that you've previously experienced, whether it's via your favorite hobby, an activity, a journey or a holiday.

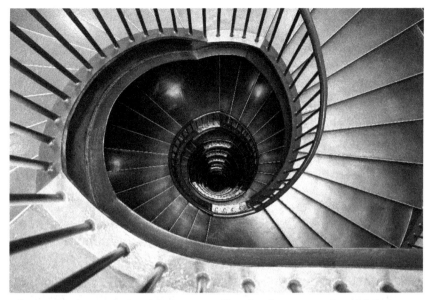

The most important thing to realize is that you should bring to your mind, relaxation, and protective magical thinking practices each day in your waking state because you know that the practice imprints it in your mind. And as time goes by, it becomes easier for you to be able to gain the benefits of these experiences, which helps to promote self-acceptance.

Once they become permanently fixed into your mind, you will experience some positive changes in your life, and they will become active by helping you to create positive changes in your life that are for your benefit, and they will lead you forward towards a real realization of those changes. And as you speak directly to the deeper inner part of the self that controls, you're eating habits and weight, you will realize that you have been eating more food than the food that your body wants or needs. And you will realize that your mind controls you're eating habits.

Now just seeing all those levers that you can adjust; you can then choose which one to use because you know that you have the power over your weight and you're eating habits. And also, you know what you're eating. The exact time and amount that you choose to eat are controlled in this place, which is the deeper part of your authentic self.

This part of the body is not your stomach or your appetite, but it controls your food, but it is your mind, and you get to ask that aspect of yourself beginning today, to develop new habits for yourself. And set new positive goals for yourself because you are laying a mental foundation for yourself, who is now a cheerful, attractive, positive, and authentic you. The great importance of this new you and your healthy, active, and attractive body is that you are eating less food, and you are happier.

The more you smile, and the more relaxed you are, the better you will look and the better you will feel. Also, you will be able to find satisfaction in eating less and pride yourself in knowing that each time you do so, you are rewarding your slimmer, healthier, and natural self. And you will know that the slimmer you are deep within you as you exercise, this new strength will grow. And as you eat healthily and sensibly, you will find yourself filling satisfied, and you will discover that the exercise makes it more reinforce and more natural towards your authentic identity.

Because it is like using and strengthening your muscles to become stronger and stronger, now eating sensibly becomes easier, easier, in a practical, and the positive way means that you are mentally asking your body the foods it needs, and then you are taking the time to listen to your own body quietly. And always check in with your body on the little food that your body needs from time to time, and you will be able to take time to integrate these ideas on a deeper level.

If you are listening to these and choosing to drift into a deeper sleep, you can just do so. Now just feeling good will allow your body to be able to drift down and go into a deeper and restful sleep. If you want to get up and continue with your activities, then you have to count from one to five, and when you reach five, you can then open your eyes and come back to the fully conscious reality.

And so, on counting one, you should allow yourself to come back to full conscious reality with relaxation and ease. Then as you count two, come back slowly to your full conscious reality, and as you count three, take some nice deep relaxing breath. Moreover, as you count four, allow your eyes to open as if you've bathed them with fresh water, and now, as you count five, open your eyes completely and adjust yourself to your environment while getting ready to carry on with your day's activity.

Remember to use words that resonate with you. The affirmations need not be empty for you. They ought to have a close relation and meaning attached to them. The proper statements for the appropriate situation goes a long way in achieving success.

You can try repeating your affirmations before you go to bed. As the brain gets ready to go on "autopilot" mode, the subconscious mind becomes more active, thereby absorbing the last bits of information for the day. Repeating affirmations before you sleep not only makes you slip into dreamland in a more confident and relaxed state but also helps to convince the mind.

You might begin to wonder why, if affirmations work, they are not used to get out of "tricky" situations. For example, if you are feeling sick, would you proceed to state, "I am cured. I am well,"? Affirmations work best with an aligned state of mind. If you believe to be well, it is more likely that you will notice a decline in symptoms. If you do not believe in your affirmations, you will continue to battle through the temperature and other physical discomforts.

Finding the right words to use can be a stroll in the park; however, remembering to repeat these words, severally could present itself as a challenge. The other obstacle you might face is having two conflicting thoughts. One of them is the carefully considered affirmation, while the other is a counterproductive negation. Try the best you can to disprove the negative thoughts but do not feed them time nor energy. It will be quite challenging to believe affirmations too at the beginning. However, as time goes on, it will become easier to convince yourself. Practice makes perfect.

Chapter 16: Preparing Your Body for Your Hypnotic Gastric Band

The physical gastric band requires a surgical procedure that involves reducing the size of your stomach pocket to accommodate a less volume of food and as a result of the stretching of the walls of the stomach, send signals to the brain that you are filled and therefore need to stop eating any further.

The hypnotic gastric band also works in the same manner, although in this case the only surgical tools you will need are your mind and your body and the great part is, you can conduct the procedure yourself. The hypnotic gastric band also conditions your mind and body to restrict excess consumption of food after very modest meals. There are three specific differences between the surgical (physical), and hypnotic gastric bands:

- In using the hypnotic band, all necessary adjustments are done by continued use of trance.
- There is an absence of physical surgery and therefore you are exposed to no risks at all.
- When compared with the surgical gastric band, the hypnotic gastric band is a lot cheaper and easier to do.

How Hypnosis Improves Communication Between Stomach and Brain

How would you know when you have had enough to eat? Initially, you will begin to feel the weight and area of the food. When your stomach is full, the food presses against and extends the stomach well, and the nerve endings in the walls of the stomach respond. When these nerves are stimulated, they transfer a signal to the brain, and we get the feeling of satiety.

Sadly, when individuals always overeat, they become desensitized to both the nerve signals and the neuropeptide signaling system. During the initial installation trance, we use hypnotic and images to re-sensitize the brain to these signs. Your hypnotic band restores the full effect of these nervous and neuropeptide messages. With the benefits of hypnotic in view, we can recalibrate this system and increase your sensitivity to these signs, so you feel full and truly satisfied when you have eaten enough to fill that little pouch at the top of your stomach.

A hypnotic gastric band causes your body to carry on precisely as if you have carried out a surgical operation. It contracts your stomach and adjusts the signals from your stomach to your brain, so you feel full rapidly. The hypnotic band uses a few uncommon attributes of hypnotic. As a matter of first importance, hypnotic permits us to talk to parts of the body and mind that are not under conscious control. Interestingly, as it might appear, in a trance, we can really convince the body to carry on distinctively even though our conscious mind has no methods for coordinating that change.

The Power of The Gastric Band

A renowned and dramatic case of the power of hypnotic to influence our bodies directly is in the emergency treatment of burns. A few doctors have used hypnotic on many occasions to accelerate and improve the recuperating of extreme injuries and to help reduce the excruciating pains for his patients. If somebody is seriously burnt, there will be damage to the tissue, and the body reacts with inflammation. The patients are hypnotized to forestall the soreness. His patients heal quite rapidly and with less scarring.

There are a lot more instances of how the mind can directly and physically influence the body. We realize that chronic stress can cause stomach ulcers, and a psychological shock can turn somebody's hair to grey color overnight. In any case, what I especially like about this aspect of hypnotism is that it is an archived case of how the mind influences the body positively and medically. It will be somewhat of a miraculous event if the body can get into a hypnotic state that can cause significant physical changes in your body. Hypnotic trance without anyone else has a profound physiological effect. The most immediate effect is that subjects discover it deeply relaxing. Interestingly, the most widely recognized perception that my customers report after I have seen them—regardless of what we have been dealing with—is that their loved ones tell them they look more youthful.

Cybernetic Loop

Your brain and body are in constant correspondence in a cybernetic loop: they continually influence one another. As the mind unwinds in a trance, so too does the body. When the body unwinds, it feels good, and it sends that message to the brain, which thus feels healthier and unwinds much more. This procedure decreases stress and makes more energy accessible to the immune system of the body. It is essential to take note that the remedial effects of hypnotic don't require tricks or amnesia. For example, burns patients realize they have been burnt, so they don't need to deny the glaring evidence of how burnt parts of their bodies are. He essentially hypnotizes them and requests that they envision cool, comfortable sensations over the burnt area. That imaginative activity changes their body's response to the burns.

The enzymes that cause inflammation are not released, and accordingly, the burn doesn't advance to a more elevated level of damage, and there is reduced pain during the healing process.

By using hypnotic and imagery, a doctor can get his patients' bodies to do things that are totally outside their conscious control. Willpower won't make these sorts of changes, but the creative mind is more grounded than the will. By using hypnotic and imagery to talk to the conscious mind, we can have a physiological effect in as little as 20 minutes. In my work, I recently had another phenomenal idea of how hypnotic can accelerate the body's normal healing process. I worked with a soldier in the special forces who experienced extreme episodes of skin inflammation (eczema). He revealed to me that the quickest recuperation he had ever made from an eczema episode was six days. I realized that the way toward healing is a natural sequence of events carried out by various systems within the body, so I hypnotized him and, while in a trance requested that his conscious mind follow precisely the same process that it regularly uses to heal his eczema, however, to do everything quicker.

One and a half days after, the eczema was gone. With hypnotic, we can enormously enhance the effect of the mind. When we fit your hypnotic gastric band, we are using the very same strategy of hypnotic correspondence to the conscious mind. We communicate to the brain with distinctive imagery, and the brain alters your body's responses, changing your physical response to food so your stomach is constricted, and you feel truly full after only a few.

What Makes the Hypnotic Work So Well?

A few people think that it is difficult to accept that trance and imagery can have such an extreme and ground-breaking effect.

Some doctors were at first distrustful and accepted that his patients more likely than not had fewer burns than was written in their medical records, because the cures he effected had all the earmarks of being close to marvelous. It took quite a long while, and numerous exceptional remedies before such work were generally understood and acknowledged.

Occasionally, the cynic and the patient are the same individuals. We need the results, but we battle to accept that it truly will work. At the conscious level, our minds are very much aware of the contrast between what we imagine and physical reality. In any case, another astounding hypnotic marvel shows that it does not make a difference what we accept at the conscious level since trance permits our mind to react to a reality that is independent of what we deliberately think. This phenomenon is classified as "trance logic."

Trance logic was first recognized 50 years ago by a renowned researcher of hypnotic named Dr. Martin Orne, who worked for a long time at the University of Pennsylvania. Dr. Orne directed various tests that demonstrated that in hypnotic, individuals could carry on as though two absolutely opposing facts were valid simultaneously. In one study, he hypnotized a few people so they couldn't see a seat he put directly before them. Then he requested that they walk straight ahead. The subjects all swerved around the seat.

Notwithstanding, when examined regarding the chair, they reported there was nothing there. They couldn't see the seat. Some of them even denied that they had served by any means. They accepted they were telling the truth when they said they couldn't see the seat, but at another level, their bodies realized it was there and moved to abstain from hitting it.

The test showed that hypnotic permits the mind to work at the same time on two separate levels, accepting two isolated, opposing things. It is possible to be hypnotized and have a hypnotic gastric band fitted but then to "know" with your conscious mind that you don't have surgical scars, and you don't have a physical gastric band embedded. Trance logic implies that a part of your mind can trust one thing, and another part can accept the direct opposite, and your mind and body can continue working, accepting that two unique things are valid. So, you will be capable to consciously realize that you have not paid a huge amount of dollars for a surgical process, but then at the deepest level of unconscious command, your body accepts that you have a gastric band and will act in like manner. Subsequently, your stomach is conditioned to signal "feeling full" to your brain after only a couple of mouthfuls. So, you feel satisfied, and you get to lose more weight.

Visualization Is Easier Than You Think

The hypnotic we use to make your gastric band uses "visualization" and "influence loaded imager." Visualization is the creation of pictures in your mind. We would all be able to do it. It is an interesting part of the reasoning. For instance, think about your front door and ask yourself which side the lock is on. To address that question, you see an image in your mind's eye. It doesn't make a difference at all how reasonable or bright the image is, it is only how your mind works, and you see as much as you have to see. Influence loaded imagery is the psychological term for genuinely significant pictures. In this process, we use pictures in the mind's eye that have emotional significance.

Although hypnotic recommendations are incredible, they are dramatically upgraded by ground-breaking images when we are communicating directly to the body. For instance, you will be unable to accelerate your heart just by telling it to beat faster. Still, if you envision remaining on a railroad line and seeing a train surging towards you, your heart accelerates pretty quickly. Your body overreacts to clear, meaningful pictures.

It doesn't make a difference whether you are listening intentionally, your conscious mind will hear all it needs to recreate the real band, in a similar way that a clear image of a moving toward train rushing towards your influences your pulse rate. You do not have to hold the pictures of the operational procedures in your conscious mind, because during an activity you are anesthetized and unconscious. Notwithstanding what you intentionally recollect, underneath the hypnotic anesthesia, your conscious mind uses this information and imagery to introduce your gastric band in the right spot.

Chapter 17: How Negative Emotions Affect Weight Loss

It appears everybody nowadays is attempting to lose weight. We are modified by our condition to look, dress, and even act in a specific way.

Each time you get a magazine, turn on the TV or check out yourself, you are reminded of it. You start to hate your body losing control, disappointed, focused on, apprehensive, and now and again even discouraged.

If losing weight is tied in with eating fewer calories than your body needs and doing some activity to support your digestion, at that point why are such a significant number of individuals as yet attempting to lose weight?

Losing weight has to do with your considerations and convictions as much as it has to do with what you eat. Give me a chance to give you a model. You are staring at the TV, and an advertisement is shown demonstrating a chocolate cheddar cake that you can make utilizing just 3 fixings. You weren't hungry previously, however, since you have seen that cheddar cake you might feel denied and you need to eat. Your feelings are revealing to you that you have to eat, although your stomach isn't disclosing to you that you are hungry.

This is called passionate eating. It is our feelings that trigger our practices.

You may find that when you are feeling focused or depressed, you have this need to eat something since it solaces you somehow or another. The issue is that generally; it isn't healthy that you get for and once you have done this a couple of times it turns into a passionate stay; so every time that you experience pressure or grief, it triggers you to eat something.

Grapples keep you attached to convictions that you have about your life and yourself that prevent you from pushing ahead. You regularly compensate yourself with things that prevent you from losing weight. When you're utilizing nourishment to reward or repay yourself, you are managing stays.

Although the grapples that I am alluding to around passionate eating are not healthy ones, they can likewise be utilized intentionally to get a specific outcome.

Enthusiastic eating doesn't happen because you are physically hungry. It occurs because something triggers a craving for nourishment. You are either intuitively or deliberately covering a hidden, enthusiastic need.

The fear of eating can assume control over your life. It expends your musings; depleting you of your vitality and self-discipline, making you separate and gorge. This will create more fear and make matters more regrettable.

So how might you conquer your fear and different feelings around eating?

You can transform the majority of your feelings around eating into another more beneficial relationship.

In all actuality, you have a soul. You should find it. It is that spot inside of you that is continually cherishing, forgiving and tranquil. It's a spot that speaks to your higher self.... the genuine you.... the sheltered, loved and entire you. When you find this, the resentment, dissatisfaction, and stress that you are feeling about your weight will vanish.

Things never appear to happen as fast as we might want them to... perhaps your body isn't changing as quickly as you need. This may demoralize you, giving you further reason to indulge.

Comprehend that your body is a gift, and afterward, you will begin to contemplate it.

Quit harping on your stomach fat, your fat arms and butt, your enormous thighs that you hate and every one of the calories that you're taking in, and see all that your body is, all that your body can do and all that your body is doing... right now.

This new mindfulness will make love and acknowledgment for your body such that you never had. You start to treasure it like the astounding gift that it is and center around giving it wellbeing every day in each moment, with each breath.

Begin concentrating on picking up wellbeing as opposed to losing weight, and you will be progressively happy, alive, and thankful. Find the delight of carrying on with a healthy life and feeding your soul consistently. Develop increasingly more love with your body and yourself, and this love will move and transform you from the inside out.

When you tap into an option that is greater than you, you have the constant motivation, which is far more dominant than any battle of the mind or feelings. Tolerating and adoring your body precisely as it is correct presently is the thing that sends the mending vibrations that will quiet your mind and transform your body from the inside out.

When you figure out how to love and acknowledge your body, you are in arrangement with your higher self, that adoring and inviting self.

Grasp what your identity is and not who you think you are or ought to be. Understand the endeavors that you make are seeds. Try not to see the majority of your efforts to lose weight as disappointments, consider them to be seeds you are planting towards progress.

Pardon yourself. Try not to thrash yourself, regardless of how frequently you think you've fizzled, irrespective of what you resemble at this moment and irrespective of how often you need that new beginning. Pardon yourself!

Emotional Weight Loss

Most overeating is emotional!

Not many people understand that they are eating for emotional reasons, and after that, follow specific problems behind their eating to attempt to cure them. If you are an overeater, you have to comprehend the reasons why you overeat, which will enable you to change your eating habits. If not, you wind up stalling out in a foolish cycle like this one; "You overeat because you're disturbed, you put on weight because you overeat, you get steamed because you've put on weight." And you never appear to break out the cycle long enough to lose weight or keep weight off.

If you have numerous pounds to lose, you must understand that your life can be such a considerable amount of superior to anything it is right at this point. If you're not content with yourself, you sure don't need to acknowledge yourself the way you are. Nobody's ideal, and we, as a whole, have problems. Everybody has something to improve in their lives, whether it's changing a harmful habit or getting more fit; the best way to accomplish is beating negative speculation by a positive attitude.

Time and again, we will, in general, discover valid justifications to justify ourselves.

For unknown reasons, many people won't concede the genuine cause of their overeating and will come up with a wide range of reasons, for example, "My parents are fat, so that's why I'm fat, it's innate." or "I have a difficult metabolism, it's so moderate." Making excuses not to eat right or exercise consistently is just a way to justifying why you can't change.

Do We Acquire Fat?

You grow up not realizing the right way to eat, and you grow up overweight. It's a decent wager that your overeating habits are indistinguishable from your folks' and that your figure much takes after theirs. What truly happens is that we acquire the terrible eating habits of those we grow up with. While obesity is once in a while genetic, it tends to be controlled by great eating habits, exercise, and a positive mental attitude.

What Is Metabolism, And How Can It Influence Your Body?

You eat food, the body at that point experiences a procedure of separating all the food and transforming it into usable energy to prop you up. To keep up a healthy weight, you have to adjust your energy IN and your energy OUT. More "in" than "out" = overweight problems. Most of us have a regularly controlled metabolism, yet many need to believe it's delayed as a reason for their weight gain. For an excessive number of people, the aftereffect of inactive living is a losing fight against those extra pounds. Through moderate day by day exercise, you will eat less and, in this manner, lose the extra pounds.

Others may state, "I can't bear to be slim."

Our general stores are loaded up with advantageous, dull plastic foods. Shopping baskets are flooded with precooked, instant, solidified foods with lost dietary benefits. These are high-cost and high-fattening foods. You can bear to eat right, and you can't manage the cost of not to!

Emotional eaters will utilize food to deal with their feelings because of food assuages pressure. When concentrating on food, it occupies our psyches from awkward feelings (fatigue, stress, tension, loneliness) that we would preferably not endure. We go after food whenever we don't like ourselves, and emotional eating turns into an imbued habit.

The initial step is to make sense of what triggers your emotional eating and figure out how to manage the stresses and stress that cause your overeating. Make sense of why you are baffled or upset and start searching for a cure to the problem. Whatever is annoying you rationally need some natural air, not a pack of chips. Work them out. Examine them with family or companions, and if you would prefer not to discuss it, accomplish something, get dynamic.

Start understanding yourself and your needs. Before going after another bit of cake, ask yourself, "Am I extremely eager?" or before you naturally pop something into your mouth, continue asking yourself, "Why am I feeling hungry?" Learn to perceive your appetite. Try not to be terrified to address yourself and get to the base of the problem.

Keep a food diary. By following you're eating habits, it will enable you to see your utilization level and comprehend what triggers your binges. Cause a rundown of different things you can do. Have a go at taking a walk, cleaning the house, working out, calling a companion or tune in to music.

Never center around dieting or weight misfortune!

If you feel wild around food, quit being fixated on your weight. Most diets expect you to boycott your preferred foods, leaving you unsatisfied and setting off negative feelings. Diet hardship sets up desires and causes you to eat more than you truly need to. Disregard dieting and spotlight on self-care, eating admirably, and being fit.

Begin concentrating on changing your lifestyle habits by eating well, practicing consistently while keeping a positive attitude. The day you quit being fixated on your weight will be the day of your prosperity. Keep in mind a specific something, you have control over your life, and it's your choice to change your lifestyle. You're justified, despite all the trouble!

Chapter 18: Weight Control Individualization

Individualization of a particular program is being stressed, and more of this is still going to happen. If you want the plan you choose to work with to be most effective and produce beautiful results, you must make it yours and ensure that it is unique to you according to what you think can work well for you. Do not start using a program that is not individualized, one that you pick from anywhere and start using because it may not work for you. As you already know, as an individual, you have a unique retinal pattern, fingerprints, and the body chemistry you have does not match that of anyone else. The things you have experienced in life are also different from those of other people.

In the same way, a program that you can use to help you in attaining a unique bodyweight should also be unique to you so that it can achieve maximum positive results. This is why you can see that here you are only provided with a few meditation exercises that you have the chance to choose the best ones that suits you. Giving you so many meditation exercises may be overwhelming when it comes to choosing the activity that suits your body and the one that you are comfortable with. When you are overwhelmed with many choices of meditation exercises to choose from, there is the possibility that you may be confused about making the right decision. Also, you can see that no meditation has been given in a stone manner, the only part that you need to put a lot of effort to ensure success is maintaining your discipline and telling yourself that you know the kind of goals you want. It would be best if you achieved them no matter what happens as you proceed with these exercises.

As an individual, you should discover which form suits you best and follow that diligently until you get the results that you aim for. Many people all over the world have tried meditation methods. Still, many of them have failed because most teachers for meditational schools believe that there is one way to meditate, which applies to each and everyone throughout the world. Many think that they have learned this method from their meditation schools and their teacher through coincidence and by being curious. But the truth is that this could be their best meditation method as individuals, but it does not mean everyone else will find it comfortable, and by using it, they must achieve success. Such kinds of people who have been disappointed because they did not get the results they expected from the meditation exercises belief that it cannot work for them, yet they have not tried other forms of meditation and see how it can work for them.

However, particular aspects come in all forms of meditational paths. For example, meditators should try to continually arrive at the maximum attention possible, which is called coherent attention in some meditational schools. This is whereby, as an individual, you decide to discipline your mind and ensure always to do one thing at a particular time to maintain focus and avoid being overwhelmed. You also decide that you love yourself, and you will treat yourself in a manner that you have promised yourself. These are some of the constants when it comes to various meditational schools. Apart from these, the other things that are involved like doing your meditation while walking in the area of your comfort, do it while sitting in an armchair, and lying on the floor are things that you should decide for yourself and consider the one that you are comfortable with. When it comes to deciding the best time for you to perform the meditational exercises; it is up to you, and there is no conventional way in which you should follow. You can choose to be doing it either once or twice in a day and perform them for one, two, or three weeks depending on what you have promised yourself that you will achieve.

As you continue, if you find that you are committed, and you have a great desire to achieve the healthy body weight that you need to have, you can decide to follow all the meditational exercises because overall, they will help you to achieve your goals. If you do not want to try different meditational paths, then you can decide to go for the combined meditations that you have explicitly identified. There are various forms of meditations that you can choose to go with. Some of these meditational paths include those that stress on the intellectual path, that those enable you to work through emotions and others that have been devised by religious groups in the western world. It does not matter the form of meditation that you have decided to use to attain your goals and experience fulfilment. The truth is that to achieve what you want with these various kinds of meditations. You must put in the work that is required. The results will not be easy for any form of meditation that you decide to go with. Be sure that whatever path you choose, you will not find any easy path because achieving the growth and development you want is difficult. The only best way to achieve what you want is that you be serious and be prepared to put an effort that will not stop soon.

These statements may seem to be put strongly, but those who have attempted to change their lives and succeeded can attest to this and tell you that it is the truth. When we work to achieve a healthy body weight through meditation, we need to know that we will not only individualize our meditational programs but also there are other aspects of our lives that we should also individualize. We will look at some of these things that we should put into consideration when it comes to individualizing the program we have.

For many years, individualization has not been taken seriously, and many have underrated it. Even some experienced psychiatrists do not seem to get it, and many of them may not understand that various patients need different help when it comes to psychotherapy. These people also need various preparedness measures to deal with impending stress due to surgery, and they should be helped differently so that they can effectively deal with allergies, grief, and other issues affecting their lives. But the modern concept does not need to incorporate this hence the reason you see why many meditations have been conditioned to think that there is a particular method of performing psychotherapy that is correct and can be used on various patients and this is the method that they learned from their teachers and mastered it carefully.

Those who try to come up with different concepts both meditation teachers and patients do not succeed in convincing others that there is a need for an individualized program for everyone for it to work well and for the patient to succeed. Many find it easy to believe that there is only one way regardless of what you are dealing with, whether it is meditation, psychotherapy, or other things that need treatment.

They do not want to face the complex situation that every one of different and the best way is to deal with each individual differently, whether this is something complicated or not. However, it would help if you got that we are different individuals with different bodies. When thinking of exercises, do not go for what has been hyped but design your individualized program because this is what can help you get the best results and follow your journey to becoming what you want to become. Are you thinking of changing the movement exercise that you have been doing? If you do not have such an exercise you are doing currently, you can add in your daily program. By looking around, try to know what is appealing to you. You can find an exercise that you are happy with. The kind of exercise you choose should be one that after you are through with the performance, you are left feeling good. If you are good with the popular exercise at the moment, you can go for it, and this could be a sweet coincidence. As you choose the exercise, you need to consider some factors like your current age, the pattern of exercises you were engaged in, and your physique. If you are okay with it, you may decide that you combine several of these exercises and add them to the specific regimen that you already have. You may choose to be jogging every morning, swimming a few laps on two days of the week, and taking a walk on days like Sundays.

As you may have already realized, the subject of the right path for each person lacking has been stressed. Meditation is also not left out, which is one of the best ways to solve various issues for some individuals. It is excellent for many great people around the world to have appreciated many people and it but remember that some people find it to be relevant and not that helpful in their lives. If you are devoted to these meditational exercises and conscientiously perform them for a period of six to eight weeks without seeing results, do not hate yourself because meditation is not your thing. By doing it, your weight cannot become worse, but even if you do not notice the benefits that you were looking for, the advantage that will be there is that you will have undertaken something that you have not done before. At the same time, you will also have engaged your mind to know various things that maybe you did not know about yourself and your body. Even when you find that meditation may not work best when it comes to solving your weight problem, the experience is benefitting, and it will help you learn a lot.

Chapter 19: The Importance of Body Confidence

Self-love is probably the best thing you can accomplish for yourself. Being infatuated with yourself furnishes you with fearlessness, self-esteem and it will by and large help you feel progressively positive. You may likewise find that it is simpler for you to experience passionate feelings for once you have figured out how to cherish yourself first. On the off chance that you can figure out how to adore yourself, you will be a lot more joyful and will figure out how to best deal with yourself paying little respect to the circumstance you are in.

Self-Confidence

Self-confidence is just the demonstration of putting a standard in oneself. Self-confidence as a person's trust in their very own capacities, limits, and decisions, or conviction that the individual in question can effectively confront everyday difficulties and requests. Believing in yourself is one of the most significant ethics to develop so as to make your mind powerful. Fearlessness likewise realizes more bliss. Regularly, when you are sure about your capacities you are more joyful because of your triumphs. When you are resting easy thinking about your abilities, the more stimulated and inspired you are to make a move and accomplish your objectives.

Meditation for Self-Confidence

Sit easily and close your eyes. Count from 1 to 5, concentrating on your breath as you breathe as it were of quiet and unwinding through your nose and breathe out totally through your mouth.

Experience yourself as progressively loose and quiet, prepared to extend your experience of certainty and prosperity right now.

Proceeding to concentrate on your breath, breathing one might say of quiet, unwinding, and breathing out totally.

In the event that you see any strain or snugness in your body, inhale into that piece of your body and as you breathe out experience yourself as progressively loose, quieter.

On the off chance that contemplations enter your psyche, just notice them, and as you breathe out to let them go, proceeding to

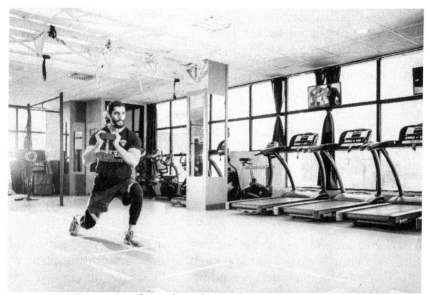

concentrate on your breath, taking in a more profound feeling of quiet and unwinding and breathing out totally.

Keep on concentrating on our breath as you enable yourself to completely loosen up your psyche and body, having a feeling of certainty and reestablishment filling your being.

Experience yourself as loose, alert and sure, completely upheld by the seat underneath you. Permitting harmony, satisfaction and certainty to fill your being at this present minute as you currently open yourself to extending your experience of harmony and happiness. And now as you experience yourself as completely present at this time, gradually and easily enable your eyes to open, feeling wide conscious, alert, better than anyone might have expected—completely present at this very moment.

Self-Love

Self-love is not just a condition of feeling better. It is a condition of gratefulness for oneself that develops from activities that help our physical, mental and profound development. Self-love is dynamic; it develops through activities that develop us. When we act in manners that grow self-love in us, we start to acknowledge much better our shortcomings just as our strengths. Self-love is imperative to living great. It impacts who you pick for a mate, the picture you anticipate at work, and how you adapt to the issues throughout your life.

There are such a significant number of methods for rehearsing self-love; it might be by taking a short outing, gifting yourself, beginning a diary or anything that may come as "riches" for you.

Meditation for Self-Love

To start with, make yourself comfortable. Lie on your back with a support under your knees and a collapsed cover behind your head, or sit easily, maybe on a reinforce or a couple collapsed covers. For extra help, do not hesitate to sit against a divider or in a seat.

In the event that you are resting, feel the association between the back of your body and the tangle. On the off chance that you are situated, protract up through your spine, widen through your collarbones, and let your hands lay on your thighs.

When you are settled, close your eyes or mollify your look and tune into your breath. Notice your breath, without attempting to transform it. What's more, see additionally on the off chance that you feel tense or loose, without attempting to change that either.

Breathe in through your nose and afterward breathe out through your mouth. Keep on taking profound, full breaths in through your nose and out through your mouth. As you inhale, become mindful of the condition of your body and the nature of your brain. Where is your body holding pressure? Do you feel shut off or shut down inwardly? Where is your brain? Is your brain calm or loaded up with fretfulness, antagonism, and uncertainty?

Give your breath a chance to turn out to be progressively smooth and easy and start to take in and out through your nose. Feel the progression of air moving into your lungs and after that pull out into the world. With each breathes out, envision you are discharging any negative considerations that might wait in your brain.

Keep on concentrating on your breath. On each breathe in, think, "I am commendable," and on each breathe out, "I am sufficient." Let each breathe in attract self-esteem and each breathe out discharge what is never again serving you. Take a couple of minutes to inhale and discuss this mantra inside. Notice how you feel as you express these words to yourself.

On the off chance that your mind meanders anytime, realize that it is all right. It is the idea of the brain to meander. Essentially take your consideration back to the breath. Notice how your musings travel in complete disorder, regardless of whether positive or negative and just enable them to pass on by like mists gliding in the sky.

Presently imagine yourself remaining before a mirror and investigate your very own eyes. What do you see? Agony and pity? Love and delight? Lack of bias?

Despite what shows up in the meditation, let yourself know: "I adore you," "You are lovely," and "You are deserving of bliss." Know that what you find in the mirror at this time might be not the same as what you see whenever you look.

Envision since you could inhale into your heart and imagine love spilling out of your hands and into your heart.

Allow this to love warm and saturate you from your heart focus, filling the remainder of your body.

Have a feeling of solace and quiet going up through your chest into your neck and head, out into your shoulders, arms, and hands, and afterward down into your ribs, tummy, pelvis, legs, and feet.

Enable a vibe of warmth to fill you from head to toe. Inhale here and realize that affection is constantly accessible for you when you need it.

When you are prepared, take a couple of all the more profound, careful breaths and after that delicately open your eyes. Sit for a couple of minutes to recognize the one of a kind encounter you had during this meditation.

Chapter 20: Hypnosis Myths

It is common to misjudge the topic of hypnotism. That is why myths and half-truths abound about this matter.

Myth: You won't recall that anything that happened when you were mesmerized when you wake up from a trance.

While amnesia may occur in uncommon cases, during mesmerizing, people more often than not recollect everything that unfolded. Mesmerizing, be that as it may, can have a significant memory impact. Posthypnotic amnesia may make an individual overlook a portion of the stuff that occurred previously or during spellbinding. This effect, be that as it may, is typically confined and impermanent.

Myth: Hypnosis can help people to recall the exact date of wrongdoing they have been seeing.

While spellbinding can be utilized to improve memory, the effects in well-known media have been significantly misrepresented. Research has discovered that trance doesn't bring about noteworthy memory improvement or precision, and entrancing may, in reality, lead to false or misshaped recollections.

Myth: You can be spellbound against your will

Spellbinding needs willful patient investment regardless of stories about people being mesmerized without their authorization.

Myth: While you are under a trance, the trance specialist has full power over your conduct.

While individuals frequently feel that their activities under trance appear to happen without their will's impact, a trance specialist can't make you act against your wants.

Myth: You might be super-solid, brisk, or physically gifted with trance.

While mesmerizing can be utilized for execution upgrade, it can't make people more grounded or more athletic than their physical abilities.

Myth: Everyone can be entranced

It is beyond the realm of imagination to expect to entrance everybody. One research shows that it is amazingly hypnotizable

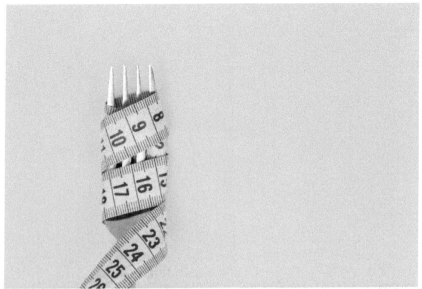

around 10 percent of the populace. While it might be attainable to spellbind the rest of the masses, they are more reluctant to be open to the activity.

Myth: You are responsible for your body during trance

Despite what you see with stage trance, you will remain aware of what you are doing and what you are being mentioned. On the off chance that you would prefer not to do anything under mesmerizing, you're not going to do it.

Myth: Hypnosis is equivalent to rest.

You may look like resting, yet during mesmerizing, you are alert. You're just in a condition of profound unwinding. Your muscles will get limp, your breathing rate will back off, and you may get sleepy.

Myth: When mesmerized, individuals can't lie,

Sleep induction isn't a truth serum in the real world. Even though during subliminal therapy, you are progressively open to a recommendation, regardless; you have through and through freedom and good judgment. Nobody can make you state anything you would prefer not to say—lie or not.

Myth: Many cell phone applications and web recordings empower self-trance, yet they are likely inadequate.

Analysts in a 2013 survey found that such instruments are not ordinarily created by an authorized trance inducer or mesmerizing association. Specialists and subliminal specialists consequently prescribe against utilizing these.

Most likely, a myth: entrancing can help you "find" lost recollections.

Even though recollections can be recouped during mesmerizing, while in a daze like a state, you might be bound to create false recollections. Along these lines, numerous trance specialists remain distrustful about memory recovery utilizing spellbinding.

The primary concern entrancing holds the stage execution generalizations, alongside clacking chickens and influential artists.

Trance, be that as it may, is a genuine remedial instrument and can be utilized for a few conditions as an elective restorative treatment. This includes the administration of a sleeping disorder, grief, and agony.

You utilize a trance specialist or subliminal specialist authorized to confide in the technique for guided trance. An organized arrangement will be made to help you accomplish your individual goals.

Chapter 21: Hypnosis may be More Effective Than Diet?

Dieting only changes the food you eat for a while and limit your mindset. Thus, Meditation will help you tap into your inner feelings and respond to your craving with the ability to control yourself.

Not being on a diet also makes you keep your focus because you will be keen on what you eat and how beneficial it is to your body. Meditation for weight loss changes the perception of the mind, which in turn triggers the inner self to respond to the choices and decisions made. Dieting is restrictive and specific on the meals you are to eat.

It challenges the mind to believe that restriction in terms of food is the only path to weight loss. Meditation, however, is a healthy way of letting the mind be free to choose what is best, learn from mistakes, and be able to focus on becoming better. It is possible to gain weight loss once one stops the diet process. It can offer both long term and short-term weight loss needs. However, the disadvantage is you must know the calories to take per serving. If you do not know, you may take less, and your body will be deprived of the needed nutrient.

Tackling Barriers to Weight Loss

There are so many barriers to weight loss from personal, to medical, to support system and emotional health. Meditation, if incorporated, will bring fruitful and healthy results. Dedication to overcome the challenges and to be focused on achieving your goals is significant. There are so many distractions, especially before you start tour weight loss routine.

It takes discipline and resilience to manage a healthy loss program. We need to give weight loss the priority it deserves. Also, we need to realize the existence of the said barriers and their contribution toward our goal. The barriers will determine our successes and failures.

Set realistic goals

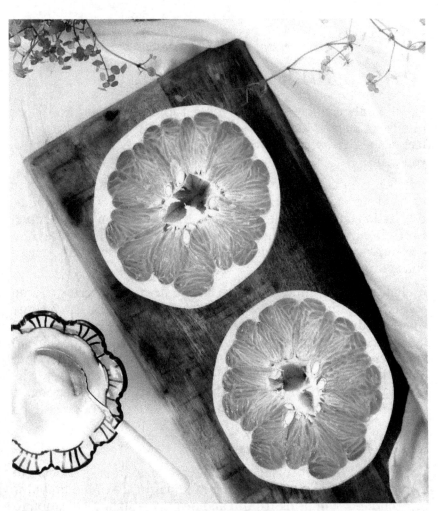

When you set goals, ensure that they are attainable, specific, and realistic. It is effortless to work on realistic goals and achieve them for better results. If the goals are unrealistic; however, the success rate will be low since on will be discouraged. For instance, when starting with meditation, you can start with as little as five minutes a day and gradually increase it daily until you reach the maximum time like sixty minutes.

The same applies to lose weight during the meditation process. You can start focusing on losing a few pounds each week and gradually increase until you reach your goal. As you set goals, however, realize that it is not your fault if they do not work out as you had planned, do your best and keep your focus.

Always be accountable

Once you have decided to commit to meditation to weight loss, don't shy away from sharing your plan with your support system and family. It is to ensure that the people you share with also reinforce the commitment and form part of the support system. That way, they will feel part of the program and give support whenever there is a need. You can also use apps for reminders and timings; this way, you have a backup plan whenever you forget.

You can also use motivational bands whenever you achieve a milestone set. Being accountable makes you enjoy your successes, acknowledge your failure, and appreciate your support system.

People thrive when they feel responsible for something, especially on something beneficial to their well-being.

Modify your mindset

Your thinking needs to be modified in the sense that you be keen on the information you are telling yourself. Ensure that your mind is not filled with unproductive and negative thoughts, which will bring you down or discourage you. Do not be scared of challenging your thoughts and appreciate your body image.

Your mindset determines your thinking, and in turn, creates a sense of appreciation or rejection. Our weight loss largely depends on our mindset. Do you believe you can do it? If you think you have all it takes, then absolutely nothing will prevent or stop you.

Manage stress regularly

Having a stress management technique should be part of one's daily routine. You need to develop a healthy stress-relieving mechanism that can help you live a stress-free life. Understand that meditation is a stress reliever in its own right as it helps calm the mind and soothes the body.

It can be used to manage stress and its benefits fully utilized to live a more productive life. Be able to handle stress efficiently. Stress is not healthy for the mind.

If not handle, it can cause emotional problems and makes one irrational, moody, or violent. Be your own boss when managing your stress.

Be educated about weight loss

As you embark on meditation for weight loss. Be educated about how it works; that way, weight loss will not be a struggle. You will be able to handle failed attempts as well as appreciate the progress made. You will be able to know what you have been doing wrong and decide on the best meditation exercise for you.

If you have misleading information, then your general progress may be inhibited

Weight loss need not be too expensive; neither does it require a costly gym membership or enrolment in a costly meditation class. There are various self-practice meditation exercises that you can comfortably do at home. There are various meal plans and diets that may work for others, though they may not offer long-term solutions or lasting behavior changes. Have the right information that you need. Don't be misled by anyone posing that they are professionals in that field. Also, do not hesitate to do research online and compare notes. From there, you will be able to come back with something that works for you.

Surround yourself with a support system

There are people out there who may be ready and willing to help whenever you want to start or even after you have started.

The support system may include your family, colleagues, friends, or social networks. These groups of amazing people may encourage and support you to meet your long-term goal. After you include them in your plan, they will feel accepted, offer opinions, and check on your progress. Analyze how things are going, as well as encourage you to continue taking a little break when necessary.

Your support system should also include professionals in the field who will give sound advice and offer needed support and care. They will also help you discover the things hindering you and holding you behind as well as offer solid information that can help you overcome. As you select the professional you want to work with, ensure they are people who are easy to talk to. People who are willing to be a participant in the routine you choose. You can also consider people who are ready to give an honest opinion as well as recommendations. Support systems sometimes have similar challenges that you may be going through at that particular time.

Their words of encouragement and best wishes usually would go a long way in motivating someone. Realize that ideologies may correspond with your point of view.

Chapter 22: How to Use Meditation and Affirmations to Lose Weight

No Nonsense Weight loss affirmations the loss of weight is a great goal, but it sure helps you to get where you want to go if you have affirmations of weight loss. So why do weight claims help you get where you want to go?

AFFIRMATION

Affirmations would help to wrap the mind around your goals and keep you focused as to where you want to be. So, when you're in its match, let's get those things moving.

Objective 1: Create the perfect healthy weight. The first bad part is to go there and achieve a certain ideal healthy weight. Don't talk about this. Even talk to your doctor about your ideal healthy level and do research. It is essential to raise an important subject at this stage. What is your ideal healthy weight and assume you can't get there? It is safe to say that when it comes to appearance and obesity, society has set some rather strict standards.

When you see it, it is quite simple to define morbid obesity. This applies to a person who struggles with everyday life while carrying out basic tasks. But what happens to all of us if these tables that describe the criteria for the ideal height, weight, and body mass index of an individual cannot be matched? What are the rules if you are too thin?

Especially if you're not fit, there is a risk of being too thin. It would be far safer to be slightly overweight, but fit and healthy according to the scale. So, use common sense and never set your ideal weight by guess or because you think that this is the only weight you can take pleasure in. Focus your ideal weight on being healthy, but above all, a weight to keep you active and fit.

Objective 2: How I Am Going to Finish Objective 1.

You have your ideal healthy weight established, and you need to get there now. It's just another wasted opportunity if you don't. Next, ignore the lazy diet pills and crash diets that will take you back to where you started or worse. How is this a positive statement? See a fat farmer ever? I say one who works the farm every day. What makes the difference? The right to eat and physical activity. The body is designed for frequent and varied exercises. The main components of Objective 2 must be both aerobic and motivational tasks. For food, a balanced diet should be consumed, which takes approximately 1800-2800 calories a day for one person and less for a woman. Include as much organic food as possible to avoid fast food and processed food. Eat vegetables and fruits.

Objective 3: Believe it!

All right, we have Target 1 and Target 2 planned, now how can we convince ourselves that we're going to achieve these without falling off the car? You've been happy to ask about this. First, why do I have to believe it? Can I not just go?

Ever hear the phrase "been there"? That could only be the case, and how did it work? Not too good, perhaps, or you wouldn't be here now.

Meet your new best friend to help you with the third objective. The meaning of these words your head doesn't know I can't, I won't give up, forget about it, or, "Let's go to the Dairy Queen," most statements are more likely to finish when they're written. Detail how your life has changed by eating better, looking better, and feeling better. Talk about where you began and how you took a step closer to achieving goal #1 each day. Talk about how you might be tempted to give up, but here you remembered, saying NOT TODAY OR EVER!! And finally, when you reach your goal, how proud you are and how you don't go the old way or weight.

Objective 4: Remember that you have your head into the game every day for goal #3. Okay, you've got to keep it in the game. How? By confirming your stated Objectives #1 to #3. You likely have to hear them out once a day so that you don't forget them. Once you free your mind, there's a saying that your rear end will lead. Hold with your head your body parts in the game.

Here are your claims of weight loss: plan it wisely, change the lifestyle, enter the game, and bring your body with you. Continue to talk to yourself because you are your best friend. This must not be torture. Take joy in the fact that the reward you want and deserve is your path.

MEDITATION

Meditation has long been recognized as the tested path to self-improvement, the ratings of which are very high because it involves only sitting there and holding your inner self and being at peace with yourself. It's a good way to change your life.

Self-esteem is one field that benefits greatly from the practice of the art of meditation. It refers to the way people view themselves, which also describes how self-confidence is nurtured.

It is believed that a daily dose of meditation will help to remove the illusion that you may have about yourself because what you are is only about how you project your image. Meditation is going to help you realize who you are.

If you have a complex of inferiority or don't think about yourself very much, it means you need to improve your image. That's where easy meditation will help you make things better; it's necessary to do your morning and evening routine. It's going to make you think better and calmer.

It is the pillar of self-esteem because it will help you have peace within yourself and increase your faith in life.

You will start interacting with people in a better way with your renewed confidence and face things with greater confidence without relying on any other support to make you feel strong.

No more pretense or attempt to pass as a character you're not going to be. This means you're going to be more comfortable and not concerned about life anymore. You're just going to relax and let life stuff take its course.

What you're going to do is take a little time every morning and night, spend no less than 30 minutes of meditation a day. You will see things start to change within two weeks or a month if you continue to do this.

Chapter 23: Psychology of Weight Loss

If you have carried on with most of your life overweight, you've in all probability attempted many weight loss programs, weight loss diets and a substantial portion of medications and pills for sure. Any individual who has experienced these encounters realizes that a definitive "diet executioner" is your very own absence of poise and core interest.

During weight loss, you can covertly be the cause of all your problems.

If you've taken a stab at losing weight or a weight loss program previously, and have observed it to be a difficult task where losing a couple of pounds to gain it all over again increasingly, then it is time that you think about what psychological cycle you go through and break out of it so you will reach your goal.

SEVEN STEPS TO BREAKING THE CYCLE

1. Stop Diet Deprivation. Diets and weight loss programs that put severe limitations on what you can eat often stimulate voraciously consuming food. While you may wait for some time, one day you'll choose to deny yourself isn't justified, despite any potential benefits, or you can't tolerate it any longer, and you dive into the more relaxed, cooler or nibble bureau furiously. Permit yourself little guilty pleasures that are fulfilling and will enable you to maintain a strategic distance from unsafe binging.

2. Plan Ahead. Imagine a scenario where you should slip. The ideal approach to abstain from slipping is through pre-planning. In this way, if you're set for a backyard grill or family assembling, choose early what your plan is. Eat something substantial and rounding before you go out and after that permit yourself a couple of rare treats at the gathering, however, exercise a bit of control. If you realize that Aunt Mary is making your preferred pastry, plan on having a little cut, and relish it. Dealing with your weight and getting a charge out of life ought to go connected at the hip.

3. Set Realistic Weight Loss Goals. To stay away from the dissatisfaction of falling flat, don't overemphasize yourself with ridiculous weight loss goals. You gained weight gradually after some time, and it will require some investment to lose that weight slowly. Slow, however, sure is the best approach.

4. Pick Healthy Outlets for Emotions. Rather than opening the fridge when you're upset, what about calling a companion, or go for a stroll? Find something that makes you feel more settled or more joyful, something other than sustenance or liquor. Do yoga, move around your front room, ruminate, or go out bowling with a companion.

5. Quit Harboring Hurts. Work through issues that are upsetting you. Converse with a specialist or even a companion. Try not to give harms, a chance to even old injuries or examples that venture back into your adolescence, influence you and your association with sustenance.

6. Keep in mind Why You're Dieting. It stops and recollects why you're dieting in any case. Is it to have more energy, look and feel better, ease medical issues, or improve your confidence? Remembering the goal is essential to your weight loss achievement.

7. Utilize Your Mind to Break the Cycle. The truth of the matter is, you can do it. It's all in your mind, the ability to lose the weight rests with you. Trust you can succeed, and you will achieve. If you need to put a conclusion to the psychological cycle of weight gain, begin by transforming the majority of your negative self-talk into positive affirmations. That is the ideal approach to break the cycle.

Rather than saying: "See that fat midsection. It just won't leave." Think positive: "Truly, my gut is fat now. However, it won't always be. I plan to be fit, not fat. I'm making a beeline for the rec center after work today."

Remember your goal consistently. Record your positive affirmations and put up visual reminders of what you need to achieve, that dress you need to purchase, that ocean side hotel you're aching to visit this year, or even an image of the cheerful individual you need to be again. It's everything inside reach if you set your mind to it, keep dynamic, exercise, and plan substantial menus that you appreciate.

Utilize these seven stages to make a psychological turnaround and move pass the psychological hindrances that are keeping you down. If you do, you'll have the ability to accomplish lasting weight loss, something that will change your future and your life.

Chapter 24: Benefits of Being Healthy to Motivate You

The process of getting that what is necessary requires you as an individual to be able to acquire some personal discipline. Before you purchase any food, you need to ask yourself if buying the food is necessary. Ask yourself if the food that you are eating will add any value to your overall health. After asking yourself that question, you will know the right thing to do based on the response to the questions. It is an easy process to do, and it will help to save you from eating those carbs that only add unnecessary weight to your body.

Maintain a healthy body

Once we consume food, our bodies respond to what we have consumed. The response could be negative or positive. Different foods generate different feelings. You may not believe what some of these feelings are, except you focus your minds on realizing them. The power of meditation is that it allows you to be able to focus, concentrate on a particular thing that requires your attention. This is an easy task to accomplish, and you only should evaluate how your body reacts to the foods that you are consuming. Once you eat some foods, you will notice that you feel energized, while some foods will make you feel tired.

Once you overeat, you will experience some sudden feelings of tiredness. You will begin to feel as if your body is too heavy, and so all you want to do is take a nap or a rest. Now when this happens, you should realize that it is a sign that whatever you ate was unnecessary, and hence the body will not use the food. As a result, most of what you ate will become something that your body needs to eliminate. Thus, you will start to add extra weight, because the excess food in your body becomes excess fat in your body. On the other hand, if once you eat, it immediately makes you feel energized; it means your body was receptive to the food that you eat.

It means that your body was able to convert much of the food into energy, and your body will well utilize each of that component

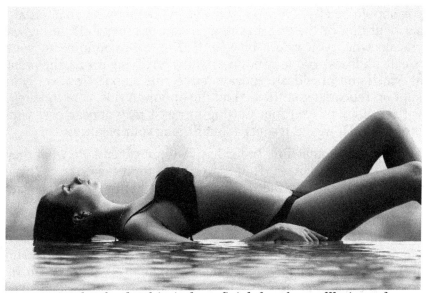

present in the food. This is beneficial for the wellbeing of your body, and it can help you when losing weight and prevent you from adding unnecessary weight.

Maintain the bodyweight

A great many people don't comprehend that adding daze to your weight reduction endeavors can enable you to lose more weight and look after it. Spellbinding originates before the tallying of carb and calories by a few decades. However, this well-established technique for centering consideration presently can't seem to be held entirely onto as an effective methodology for weight reduction.

As of not long ago, the real claims of prestigious trance inducers have been bolstered by insufficient logical proof, and an excess of pie in the sky responsibilities from their issue kin, stage trance specialists, have not made a difference.

Seeing is thinking absolutely. So, investigate yourself. To gain proficiency with a portion of the priceless exercises that trance must instruct about weight reduction, you don't need to be spellbound. The ten smaller than expected ideas that pursue contain a portion of the eating regimen modifying recommendations that my gathering and individual hypnotherapy weight the executive's clients get.

The power is inside. Trance specialists believe that you have all you should be effective. You truly needn't bother with an alternate accident diet or the ongoing suppressant of hunger. Thinning, as you do when you ride a bike, is tied in with confiding in your innate abilities. You may not recall how terrifying it was, the point at which you previously endeavored to ride a bike. However, you kept on rehearsing until you had the option to ride, consequently, with no idea or exertion. Getting more fit may appear past you, moreover. However, it's just about finding your balance.

You see your conviction. Individuals will, in general, do what they accept they can achieve. That is even valid for mesmerizing. Those fooled into deduction they could be entranced (for example, as the trance inducer proposed they would see red, he turned the switch on a disguised red bulb) demonstrated improved mesmerizing reaction. It is essential to hope to be made a difference. Give me a chance to propose you anticipate that your arrangement should work on weight reduction. Highlight the positive. Recommendations, for example, "Doughnuts will sicken you," negative or aversive, work for some time, however on the off chance that you need lasting change, you need to think emphatically. Specialists Herbert Spiegel and David Spiegel, a dad child hypnotherapy group, considered the most well-known valuable trance-like proposition. "I need my body to live in. I owe regard and security to my body." I elevate clients to create their very own energetic mantras. A 50-year-old mother who shed 50 pounds more rehashes day by day: "Superfluous nourishment is a weight on my body. I will shed what I needn't bother with."

It's going to come if you envision it. Like competitors who are getting ready for the challenge, you are set up for a successful truth by picturing triumph. Envisioning a smart dieting day will enable you to envision the means expected to turn into a decent eater. Is it too difficult to even think about photographing? Locate a comfortable old photograph of yourself and recall what you did another way. Envision these schedules reviving. Or, on the other hand, picture acquiring direction from a more former, more astute self later on in the wake of contacting her required weight.

Get rid of cravings. Subliminal specialists utilize the intensity of emblematic symbolism on a standard premise, welcoming subjects to put sustenance desires on fleecy white mists or inflatables in sightseeing and send them up, up, and away. On the off chance that you can direct off your eating routine from McDonald's brilliant curves, trance inducers comprehend that a counter-image can control you back. Welcome your psyche to flip through its picture Rolodex until you develop as an indication of yearnings throwing out. Push.

There are two preferred procedures over one. A triumphant mix is entrancing and Cognitive Behavioral Treatment (CBT) with regards to getting more fit and holding it off, which patches up counterproductive thoughts and practices. Clients learning both lose twice as much weight without falling a few, recuperate more trap of the health food nut. On the off chance that you've at any point kept up a sustenance journal, you've officially endeavored CBT. They monitor everything that experiences their lips for possibly 14 days before my clients learn mesmerizing. Each great trance inducer comprehends that raising cognizance is a principle move for the tyke towards suffering change.

Modify and then change. The late pioneer of spellbinding, Milton Erickson, MD, focused on u's essentialness. To improve the lose-recuperation, the lose-recuperation example of one customer, Erickson recommended that she put on weight first before losing it—an intense sell today, except if you're Charlize Theron. Simpler to swallow: Modify your craving for high calories.

Like it or not, it is the fittest for survival. No proposal is sufficiently able to supersede the nature of survival. Similarly, as we like to believe, it's the most appropriate survival, despite everything we're modified for survival in case of starvation. A valid example: a private dietary mentor needed a proposal for her dependence on a sticky bear. The advisor attempted to clarify that her body felt that her life relied upon the chewy desserts and wouldn't surrender them until she got enough calories from progressively nutritious food. No, she demanded, all that she required was a proposition when she dropped out.

Practice makes perfect. There are no washboard abs delivered by one Pilates class, and one spellbinding session can't shape you're eating routine. Be that as it may, discreetly rehashing a useful suggestion 15 to 20 minutes every day can change your eating, especially when combined with moderate, regular breaths, the foundation of any program of social change.

Improved mental functioning

This practice is exceptionally similar to the old practice, only instead of merely visualizing the room you want to describe it to yourself. Imagine as though you are mentally chatting with yourself or someone else and explain what the room looks like as you go about doing it. Say, for example, "The room has white walls, a white door, and white framing around the door. It has a green chair in the corner, a white desk on the north-facing wall, and a window that faces the East."

You want to describe this room down to the minutest detail you can recall for that room. Do not skip on details, describe everything you can recall. The idea is that you want to complete this exercise while also improving your attention and mental awareness. As you do this, you will be engaging in both visualization and verbalization, which can be helpful to those who are not entirely visually oriented. You can also describe the details out loud if you feel that you need even more of a verbal to your practice.

If you are not someone who prefers to use movement to enter your trance-like state but would rather do so by remaining still and calm within yourself, then you can try taking advantage of visualization. Visualization is a great practice that allows you to take control of your mind's eye and "leave" your physical body by entering your mind, instead. The following visualization practice is a great way to get your mind in control and enter a trance-like state so that you can begin your self-hypnosis practice.

Get into a comfortable position and then let your eyes fall closed. Once they have, consider a room that you are used to entering. It can be any room that you know well, and that helps you feel comfortable.

Once you have considered the room, begin to visualize it. You want to place as many details into that room as possible. Consider the colors of the walls, the door frame, the door itself, and any windows that might be in that room. Consider the view you get on the outside of the window and then visualize all the contents of the room. All the furniture, decorations, and other objects that fill the room should be "built" into your visualized version of this room.

Now, consider the differences between the two experiences. Notice how well you were able to mentally design the first room and your discrepancies in the second room. As you do, also notice how deep of a relaxation you have entered and use that to help you relax further. Then you can begin practicing your self-hypnosis practices.

Chapter 25: Eating Healthy to Keep Up with Proper Nutrition

Eating Healthy Vs. Achieving Your Goal Physique

With the idea of attaining a fantastic body, folks instantly consider eating healthy. Nevertheless, eating healthy foods does not automatically mean that you're achieving your target body. While obtaining your very best body does not exactly mean that you're eating healthy. To eat healthily means typically you give your body with sufficient nutrients to operate effectively. Your body needs a particular number of micronutrients (vitamins and minerals) and macronutrients (carbohydrates, proteins, and carbohydrates) to work in its very best ability. You must satisfy your body's nutrient requirements to keep decent health. Reaching a fantastic body usually involves losing weight or gaining muscle. To be able to lose excess weight, a person must maintain a calorie deficit wherever your body burns off more calories than the number of calories you eat and drink. Gaining weight requires you to do the contrary, at which in a calorie excess you have more calories than the amount the body burns off calories off.

Though eating healthful foods has unlimited benefits, it's just as important to satisfy the necessity of attaining your exercise goal. By way of example, if your objective is to burn fat and you also eat 10,000 calories worth of veggies every day, you are eating healthy but are consuming a lot of calories to achieve your objective. Because of this, it's best to consume towards your target body when keeping excellent health.

What's a Calorie?

You hear about calories all the time, but what does it mean? A calorie is a device that measures energy. The food that you eat is not measured in size or weight, but by how much energy it's. If you hear something that includes 100 calories, it is a method of describing just how much energy your body might gain from drinking or eating it. As the quantity of gas pumped into a vehicle is measured in gallons, different food, or beverages you eat is measured in calories. The body breaks down food in an

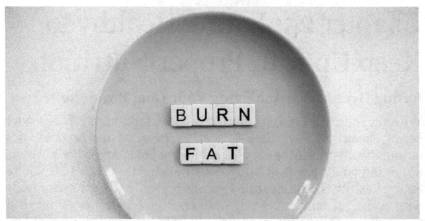

exceptional manner, so the number of calories is a means of understanding how much energy your system will get from whatever you eat or drink. 'Calorie' is only a specialized phrase for 'energy'.

Are Calories Bad for You?

Calories aren't bad for you because the body needs them to get energy. Nevertheless, eating a lot of calories and not burning off enough of these off through physical activity may cause weight gain with time. Consuming too small calories over time won't enable your body to work properly and may harm your wellbeing. Foods like lettuce contain hardly any calories (1 cup of shredded lettuce has less than ten calories). In contrast, foods such as peanuts have plenty of calories (1/2 cup of peanuts contains 427 calories daily). Understanding how many calories your body requires each day can allow you to select which foods are right for you.

How Does Your Body Use Calories?

Your body requires calories simply to remain alive and function properly. This energy is utilized for basic functions like maintaining your heart beating and lung breathing. Calories are crucial for several fundamental and intricate functions such as the regulation of body temperature as well as also the functioning of each cell in the human entire body. The more activity you do will be that the more calories you burn off. Your body also requires calories to grow and grow. You burn calories before considering it as during the digestion of food, recovery of muscles after exercise, as well as while you are sleeping.

How Many Calories Do You Want?

Folks differ in size and have different metabolisms; therefore, the number of calories an individual should eat will change based upon many things. These factors include an individual's height, age, weight, and daily activity level. The larger an individual is, the more calories a person could want, vice versa. Although two individuals can have exactly the identical body dimensions, the number of calories that they want can differ due to the way their body adjusts exactly what they eat. Calorie calculators are available on the internet, which may be employed to ascertain the number of calories your body requires depends on the vital facets. If you consume many calories than your body wants, then the additional calories are converted to fat. If you consume fewer calories than you require, then your system uses your stored body fat as the energy it needs to function. Knowing the number of calories, you want can allow you to control your weight.

Macro Basics

Macronutrients or macros are carbs, fats, and protein. Together with the expression "macro," meaning quite big, these three nutrients are responsible for supplying calories (the only other material that supplies calories is alcohol, however, isn't a macronutrient because we don't want it for survival). Whatever that you eat is broken down into those three macronutrients. Your body doesn't recognize the food that you consume as "poultry, sausage, rice, etc." Rather, your entire body sees anything you eat as a carbohydrate, fat, or protein. This is why you find these macronutrients written in bold letters to the nutrition label of any food or beverage product.

What's a Carb?

Carbohydrate is the body's main source of energy. There are two kinds of carbohydrates, complex and simple. A very simple carbohydrate supplies your body with rapid energy but does not last long. An intricate carbohydrate takes more time to break down on your body; nevertheless, it is a long-lasting supply of energy. Neither simple nor complex carbohydrate is bad for you. They could both be utilized to your benefit throughout the day. Upon waking in the morning, you likely have not had anything to eat for the past couple of hours since you have been asleep. Therefore, it is sometimes a fantastic idea to eat simple carbohydrates for instant energy. If you intend on being from home for a couple of hours, complex carbohydrates are a great selection for its long-term steady energy. So, integrating both kinds of carbohydrates in your diet may permit you better to manage your levels of energy throughout the day.

Examples of complex carbohydrates include whole grains like whole Wheat bread, oatmeal, and brown rice alongside other foods like sweet potato and beans. Simple carbs include foods like fruits, white bread, white rice, white potatoes, veggies, juice, pop tarts, etc. Sugar is a simple carbohydrate that comes in various forms like sugar, fructose, lactose, sucrose, etc. Though both intricate and straightforward carbohydrates are broken down to glucose within the body, absorption and digestion are the principal differences between both different types.

What Is Protein?

Protein helps build and repair tissue when playing a role in various cell functions within the body. It's a significant element for growing nails, hair, muscle, and different areas of the human body. Amino acids are building blocks of protein. An entire protein includes all 20 amino acids, even while the lack of one or more amino acids is known as an incomplete protein. Complete proteins are primarily found in meats like poultry, beef, beef, and fish in addition to legumes, milk, and whey protein. Foods like grains, seeds, nuts, or beans are considered incomplete proteins. It's encouraged to eat at least 0.8 - 1.2 g of protein per 1 pound of your body weight for optimum muscle development. With several unique forms of protein in the marketplace which range from the origin, absorption rate, and procedure of filtration, any comprehensive protein is helpful for the growth and repair of muscle. Poultry, fish, milk, legume, soy, whey, and other resources of proteins have their differences, but any comprehensive protein is of fantastic advantage for repairing and building muscle. The crucial thing is to find sufficient protein to satisfy your body's need for optimum growth.

What Is Fat?

Fat controls hormones, aides from the transportation of cells, and makes it feasible for different nutrients to finish tasks within the body. Fat can also be your body's secondary source of vitality. When your body doesn't have sufficient carbohydrates easily available, it uses fat as an alternative source of gas. As a result, the notion of burning fat is to limit the quantity of primary energy (carbohydrates) so the body can utilize its secondary resource of energy (body fat). Various kinds of fats contain saturated fat, polyunsaturated, monounsaturated, and trans-fat. It's encouraged to steer clear of trans-fat because of its health advantages. While every kind of fat has its advantages and disadvantages, it's helpful to look closely at the whole amount of fat in a single product.

Foods that have a high number of fat include peanut butter, oils, avocado, and nuts. Consuming low levels of fat over the years may lead to hormone levels to become erratic, which makes it important to have enough even while attempting to burn off fat. The quantity of fat required daily could vary anywhere from 15 percent to over 40 percent of total calories based on the person and fitness target.

Quality of Weight Loss or Weight Gain

If you're in a calorie deficit where your body burns off more calories than you eat, then you are going to eliminate weight. This doesn't automatically make sure that the entire weight you lose is only going to come from fat. Your body is composed of lean mass, fat, and fat. This implies any weight that's lost or obtained may come from any one of those three. When shedding fat, you risk losing weight, and if gaining weight, you risk placing on excess fat. Not monitoring macros puts you at a greater risk for muscle loss and fat gain since you would not understand how many calories you're becoming. Consuming the ideal amount of protein, fat, and carbohydrates helps to make sure you keep muscle while shedding weight and restrict the rise of body fat while incorporating muscle.

More Energy, Better Mood

Carbohydrates are the body's most important source of energy, therefore getting too little carbohydrates over time may leave you feeling exhausted and contribute to inadequate workout functionality. By properly setting up your macros, you optimize the number of carbohydrates you can consume while burning off fat. If you may eat more food while losing weight, then why not make the most of fat is in charge of controlling your hormones, therefore not having sufficient can lead to an imbalance that could result in mood swings and other undesirable symptoms. It's normal to drop short of your everyday fat requirements by merely eating "clean" foods that typically include little to no fat. Consuming low fat and carbohydrates over time may allow you to feel exceptionally miserable. To believe losing weight is a struggle, why make it tougher on yourself to accomplish your objective.

Chapter 26: The Practice of BioBalancing

This is your life. This moment. Here and now. The place you want to be is here and now. The person you want to be is right here, right now. The best that life has to offer isn't somewhere else. Life can only be lived right where you are, at this moment. But the question is... is your mind present here and now?

The reason I ask is that the act of BioBalancing is a very mindful skill. BioBalancing is like an anchor into the present moment. Each time you check-in with yourself, you are mindful. Each time you cater to your needs, you are displaying the mindful traits of compassion and love. This can have a powerfully positive knock-on effect for the rest of your life.

This is how this works:

The more you practice BioBalancing, the more clarity and understanding you'll have of your internal emotional landscape. It motivates and drives you to your desire. Your true needs and wants to become apparent. Your core values become more defined. You won't get some glaring flashing sign or signal, it's much subtler than that, just a general feeling of when something is "right" and when something is "wrong" for you—a sort of deep sense of wisdom. You'll know, deep in your soul. Once you get a clearer indication of what makes you happy, you can start to align your life accordingly to achieve more of it.

I believe this is the secret key to true happiness. It's not about getting more stuff, a bigger house or a fancier car. It's about you tapping into the real you and discovering what makes you truly fulfilled and happy. It's what we all want deep down. To live a happy life. To experience that true happiness that sinks deep into your bones and effects everything you do.

To do this, follow the 3 BioBalance principles:

1. Nourish: Ensure you are addressing your core needs.

2. Observe: Observe your emotional landscape within your body and discover what's important to you.

3. Rebalance: Figure out what you need to do to achieve more of what you want at a deeper level.

You know, recently I've become passionate about taking my family out for walks. I love staring at the scenery, watching the grass, feeling the wind and just being amazed. That abundance, that feeling of life, it's blissful. This is something I have discovered I enjoy from tapping into my body's sense.

My life has changed in so many positive ways since I started listening to my internal guidance system. That's not to say my life is all sunshine and roses, it still certainly has its fair share of challenges, but when you're connected to the true you, when you're feeling balanced and when you nourish your core needs, life flows a lot smoother. A profound shift occurs in how you feel, in how you interact with others, in your relationships, your sense of self, your productivity. Everything.

Balance NOT perfection

What you need to keep in mind is that we're striving for a more balanced life, not a perfect life (perfection doesn't exist, and it's a sure-fire path to misery). The keyword is "striving". We are never, ever, truly perfectly balanced. Like a tree blowing in the wind, we need to allow ourselves to sway from side to side when the wind blows. Our life needs to be flexible, and we need to be open to and accepting of whatever crops up in the present moment. Life can throw us a curveball at any moment, and we need to be ready to accept that. The key is to have an attitude of always striving for balance while becoming more accepting of unexpected changes and outcomes (this includes setbacks and relapses!).

So, learn to trust your inner wisdom, your instincts, and your body awareness. If it feels right for you, it is right for you. If it doesn't feel right, then change it. All the wisdom and knowledge you need is already there, inside you.

The great thing about BioBalancing is that it is a skill. It's something you can get better throughout your life. It is a process of self-discovery in the truest sense. It's a wonderful journey of self-exploration, and it helps to strengthen, nurture and enhance the most important relationship in your life: The one you have with yourself.

Chapter 27: A New Self

Validation: Seek, and You Shall Find

Your new belief is extremely fragile until it gets locked into your identity or part of your construct of the world. You closed in your old limiting beliefs, ingraining them into your psychology, by validating them over and over again. In the same fashion—but consciously, this time—you can now make these new beliefs "real" to you.

Its job is to recognize and find everything within your environment that you have predetermined to be vital to you. It begins to find everything that lines up with what you expect to see, specifically, what matches your beliefs. That's why you don't notice something—the car or purse you finally purchased, the type of house you chose to live in, a particular piece of jewelry that interests you—until it becomes somehow important to you.

All of a sudden, it's almost magically everywhere.

That's how you find what you're looking for. There was a point when building our speaking center suite in Northern California when my wife and the designers started to drive me to every flooring company in the area. It seemed like the goal was for me to see every possible option of granite, travertine, limestone, hardwood, and carpeting. Apart from being fascinated at how many flooring companies seemed to pop up in town suddenly, I'm amazed at how I still can't drive by and not notice them. Even though it's been years, I can't help but see them in the corner of my eye when I drive by. The stores had always been there; they were just "invisible" until they became important to me.

Your new belief needs to become a top priority on your "Importance List"—the things your brain is selectively looking out for. Remember that your brain craves consistency in your interpretation of the matrix of the world. It's always making sure that it's validating your construct of beliefs. Whenever there's a discrepancy, that's a chance for growth and an opening for a new belief. Building up the much-needed evidence for your new belief will allow your brain to make this belief a reality.

Familiarity Breeds Identity

Remember that, according to the well-respected developmental biologist Bruce Lipton, up to 95% of our behavior is unconscious.

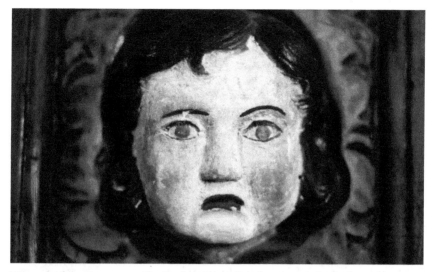

You are less in control of what you do than you thought you were. Remember that our emotions pull the strings of our behavior. Look back at your day to day; how many of your decisions were made on autopilot? Did you brush your teeth the same way, using the same toothpaste, bought from the same store as always? Did you drink the same coffee, the same way as you always do? Did you drive the same route to get to your usual destination? When you first turned on your computer, did you visit the same favorite sites?

I'm not saying this is good or bad. I'm not passing judgment. I'm saying it's important to raise your awareness of this because you create your habits, and then your habits create you. Behavioral scientists, neuroscientists, and psychologists are in general agreement that it's the repetition of the same habitual patterns of thoughts, feelings, and behaviors that create your identity. Your past conditioned your old patterns. This is your blueprint, and it's your current wiring; it's how you do things because it's how you are. This is what makes change so hard. To leave the security and certainty of your old self can be uncomfortable and daunting.

That's when most will back out. They'll revert to what they know. They'll cave in and give up.

The solution is to stop living in the past. You can't create a different future otherwise. Change happens the moment your mind stops living in the conditioned programs of the past and starts living for the future.

Chapter 28: Goal Setting

For many bariatric patients, goals are not a foreign concept. You've likely worked on your weight loss goals long before you ever thought about surgery as an option.

You likely know what your goals are. Yet, you are probably cynical, since up until now, it's been hard to reach them. Following bariatric surgery, it gets more comfortable because you see the amazing progress and you see it quickly. There are stalls in weight which can freak people out.

"Am I stuck? Will I continue to lose? Is this a plateau? How long will I be here (at this weight)?"

The panic sets in.

First, calm down. If you are doing what needs to be done, your weight will continue to drop. As you lose weight, your body is adjusting to a sharp decrease in food intake. You may want to discuss with your surgical team (bariatrician, dietician, etc.) Regarding how many calories you are getting and whether you need to decrease or increase your caloric intake.

You may be shocked at this, but sometimes the reason people are not losing weight is that they are simply not eating enough, and the body has engaged in starvation mode, so it is hanging on to every morsel in your body. Other times, you may need to reduce your calories to continue to experience weight loss. This is a very personal issue, and stalls do happen.

We all experience them. Some people experience stalls that last two weeks and some people experience stalls that last six weeks. This is when it's important to reach out to your physician or dietitian to evaluate what you may or may not be doing to help you drop. This is why awareness is essential. If you are eating off-plan and not aware, you're returning to autopilot behavior that may be causing you to gain the weight.

Another study found that when people were engaged in self-monitoring, they did a better job of losing weight and keeping the weight off (Odom et al., 2009). Self-monitoring consists of keeping a food journal, tracking exercise and other progress, as well as tracking water intake, supplements, and emotions.

It's a good idea to grab a food journal to track you're eating on a

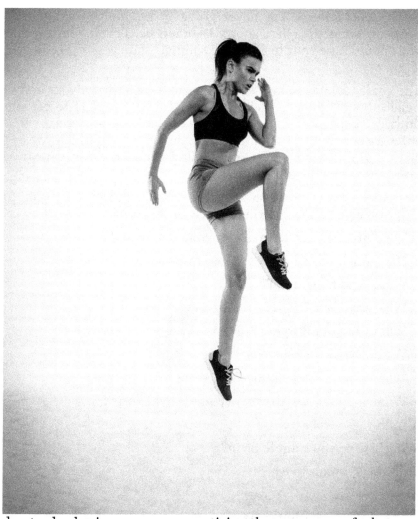

day-to-day basis, so you are practicing the awareness of what you are eating. This helps you consciously process what you are about to put into your mouth or reflect on what you already ate on any given day. It's been shown that when you are more conscious of your choices, you make better ones.

It is important to be realistic about your goals, and it's essential that you discuss this with your surgeon as well. I also need to note here; for some individuals, the BMI chart can be deceiving.

This does not mean you get a free pass to bypass the BMI chart. However, it's important to see where you fall and whether it's a factor in your actual body fat percentage overall. As someone who is 5'11 tall, I know I'm never going to be 160lbs, and that is precisely what the chart shows I should be. I'm not saying that you should hide your head in the sand, or state you're 'big-boned' if you're not.

The goal is for you to lose weight and to be healthy for your body's height. It's all about proportion. The goal here is NOT to get you down to a specific weight per se, but to get you to a weight that YOU are comfortable at, and at a weight and size in which you feel good living in your body. You, feeling comfortable in your own body, makes all the difference.

Let's look at your personal goals for short-term and long-term, to help you gain an idea of where you want to be.

~ What are the realistic goals for your weight and height?

~ How much do you expect to lose overall?

~ What is your HEIGHT?

~ What was your HIGHEST weight?

~ What was your Surgery Weight?

~ What is your Current Weight?

~ What is your ideal ending Goal Weight?

~ What are your post-surgery (pounds lost) goals for:

Month 1:

What size do you want to be in?

How do you want to feel?

Month 3:

What size do you want to be in?

How do you want to feel?

Month 6:

What size do you want to be in?

How do you want to feel?

Month 9:

What size do you want to be in?

How do you want to feel?

Month 12:

What size do you want to be in?

How do you want to feel?

Month 18:

What size do you want to be in?

How do you want to feel?

Month 24:

What size do you want to be in?

How do you want to feel?

Month 30:

What size do you want to be in?

How do you want to feel?

Month 36:

What size do you want to be in?

How do you want to feel?

If you don't know what you want, how will you go after it?

Clarity is so important. Knowing what you want is step one. If you do not yet know what you will do once you lose the weight, start thinking about it now.

The plan is to lose weight and to do all the things you have not had the opportunity to do as an obese individual. There's so much more life for you to live and many things that I know you want to do.

~ Do you have a desire to travel to Europe and walk through the ancient streets of Rome?

~ Do you want to walk/run a 5k?

~ Do you want to chase after your grandchildren and be able to pick them up at a moment's notice?

~ Or would you like to feel comfortable making love to your husband/wife?

~ What is it that means the most to you?

~ What are those things that you're excited to do now that you're losing the weight?

List them out.

Chapter 29: Find Your Motivation

One of the tools that are powerful in creating a significant change in life is Motivation. Your Motivation is based on what you believe. And as you are probably aware, belief is scarcely based on your concrete reality. In essence, you think things because of how you see them, feel them, hear them, smell them, and so forth. You can program your mind by taking feelings from one of your experiences and connecting those feelings to a different experience. Let us look at how you can remain motivated to lose weight:

Establish where you are now

It would be best if you took a full-length picture of yourself at present as a push mechanism from your current position, as well as for comparison later on. Two primary factors are relevant to health. One is whether you like the image you see in the mirror, and the second is how you feel. Do you have the energy to do what you wish and are you feeling strong enough?

· Explore your reasons for wanting to lose weight. These are what will keep you going even when you don't feel like it.

· Assess your eating habits and establish your reasons for overeating or indulging in the wrong foods.

· It is assumed that you have the desire to get healthier and lose weight. Here, you state clearly and positively to yourself what you want, and then decide that you will accomplish it with persistence. Use the self-hypnosis routine explained above to drive this point into your subconscious mind.

· Determine your Motivation for the desired results, and how you will know when you've accomplished the goal. How will you feel, what you will see, and what are you likely to hear when you achieve your goal?

· Devote the first session of self-hypnosis to making the ultimate decision about your weight. Note that you must never have any doubt in your mind about your challenge to lose weight. Plan your meals every day. Weigh yourself frequently to monitor your progress as well. However, do not be paranoid about weighing yourself as this can negatively affect your development.

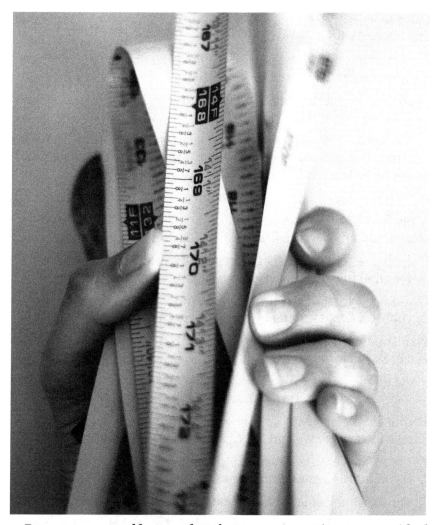

· Repeat to yourself every day that you are getting to your ideal weight, that you've developed new, sensible eating habits, and that you are no longer prone to temptation.

· Think positively and provide positive affirmations in your self-induced hypnotic state.

Tweak Your Lifestyle

Every little thing counts. This lesson is essential to know if you want to lose weight and slim down. Making a few changes in your regular daily activities can help you burn more calories.

Walk more

Use the stairs instead of the escalator or elevator if you're going up or down a floor or two.

Park the car you use far away from your destination and walk the rest of the way. You can also walk briskly to burn more calories.

During your rest day, make it more active by taking your dog for a long walk in the park.

If you need to travel a few blocks, save gas and avoid traffic by walking. For greater distances, dust off that old bike and pedal your way to your destination.

Watch how and what you eat.

A big breakfast kicks your body into hypermetabolism mode so you should not skip the first meal of the day.

Brushing after a meal signals your brain that you've finished eating, making you crave less until your next scheduled meal.

If you need to get food from a restaurant, make your order to-go so you won't get tempted by their other offerings.

Plan your meals for the week, so you can count how many calories you are consuming in a day.

Make quick, healthy meals, so you save time. There are thousands of recipes out there. Do some research.

Eat inside a place with a table, not in your car. Drive-thru food is almost always greasy and full of unhealthy carbohydrates.

Put more leaves, like arugula and alfalfa sprouts on your meals to give you more fiber and make you eat less.

Order the smallest meal size if you need to eat fast food.

Start your meal with a vegetable salad. Dip the mixture into the dressing instead of pouring it on.

For a midnight snack, munch on protein bars or drink a glass of skim milk.

Eat before you go to the grocery to keep yourself from being tempted by food items that you don't plan to buy.

Clean out your pantry by taking out food items that won't help you with your fitness goals.

The whole idea in the tweaks mentioned is that you should eat less and move more.

Chapter 30: The Conditions of Manifesting

The 8 Conditions of Manifesting

How to begin the process of manifesting.

Now, how to will it be given.

Step 1:

You've discovered this fantastic idea called the Law of Attraction, which promises "all of your dreams can become a reality. "Everything is getting more exciting. You perform a basic Google search for "how to manifest" or some similar search term. What do you find? Approximately 200 million results! The most common formula presented is one coined from popular books and the movie, The Secret, all which suggest there are three simple steps to the Law of Attraction.

Countless listings suggest you can use "7 steps to manifest anything you want"—or maybe 5 or 4. Perhaps, you'll see "how to manifest overnight" or "manifest instantly." The options go on... and on. The list of formulas, processes, systems, step-by-step strategies is endless. Each promotes a similar thinking strategy, "follow these steps in this particular order, and all your dreams will come true."

Step 2:

Figure out which one of these approaches makes the most sense for you and start following each step.

Step 3:

After anywhere from 1-to-7 days, to even God forbid, 30 days or more trying to manifest what you want, you find yourself in a dilemma. There you sit still trying to manifest what you want. Now you're thinking, "Yup, just like I thought all along, the Law of Attraction doesn't work!" Sound familiar?

Yet, somewhere deep inside you, you still long to believe. This stuff is out there for a reason so being resilient; you get up, dust yourself off, and try again—even harder this time. And again, you fail to get the results you want! Now you have double the data and double the discouragement.

What happened?

Here's the deal. While each of these approaches has some truth to them, the strategy is somewhat flawed, when presented as a linear, step-by-step process.

The Law of Attraction is not a step-by-step, one-size-fits-all process, and it's not linear.

A linear process is something that progresses directly from one stage to another with a starting point and an ending point.

LOA is most often described as a process because it's easier to explain and market the concept that way.

I'm willing to risk going against all those other processes to share the truth from my experience. The Law of Attraction is a bit messier than what's popularly suggested. If you want to make it work, I suggest following good old Einstein's wise words, "If you want different results, you have to try different approaches."

My experiences show that manifesting is best described in non-linear terms. I say it does not progress or advance like phases, going in some logical sequence. Rather, "Law of Attraction is when the manifesting conditions and personal qualities are developed and come into alignment simultaneously."

Each condition plays an important role in manifesting. And they do not always happen in the order in which they will appear in this text. These conditions can all be in play at once.

Law of Attraction is about being in alignment with all eight of the manifesting conditions, simultaneously.

The "formula," if you will, is to work through each of the conditions for manifesting only. By doing this, you will gain an understanding of what it means to be in alignment with that condition. Be sure to do the exercise assignments to support your endeavor further.

Think of it a little like juggling eight balls at a time. Start by getting good at juggling the one ball. Then add a second, and a third. With practice, soon, you will learn to juggle all eight balls at once. This is when you are in alignment with your manifestation.

The time it takes is the time it takes. Seriously! You can be in alignment with all eight conditions within a matter of a second, or it can take 20 years. It all depends on how quickly or slowly you get into alignment with each condition. But the moment you are in alignment, a manifestation is instant.

The Manifesting Conditions:

Condition #1 Desire

Defined: A strong feeling of wanting to have something or wishing for something to happen.

Condition #2 Thought

Defined: An idea or opinion produced by thinking or occurring suddenly in the mind.

Condition #3 Imagination

Defined: The formation of a mental image of something. Form a mental picture of; imagine.

Condition #4 Belief/Expectancy

Defined: Accept as real; feel sure of the truth of.

Condition #5 Feeling/Vibration

Defined: An emotional state or reaction.

Condition #6 Creative Attraction

Defined: The action or power of drawing forth a response: an attractive quality.

Condition #7 Inspired Action

Defined: The process of doing something, arising from creative impulse, to achieve something extraordinary.

Condition #8 Manifestation

Defined: To make evident or certain by showing or displaying.

Chapter 31: Overcome Your Weight Loss Plateau

There's no room for error when you set yourself up with strict, black and white guidelines to abstain entirely from those foods. You are on or off the diet, either. You're off the wagon once you've had the cookie—and that means anything goes. What's the difference between two and twelve cookies? Next week you will continue the sugar ban again—or probably next month.

Here's the worst part: the guilt, embarrassment, and self-criticism resulting from "breaking the rules" that prevent you from making reasonable efforts. It may sound like self-sabotage, but it's very logical in fact: if you realize you're punishing yourself for failure, why try? Who needs punishment? In our curriculum, we refer to ourselves as the Inner Critic, the self-critical element. It's a cruel inner voice that focuses on only one part of ourselves—such as a sugar weakness—with a meanness heart, without looking at the bigger picture of who we are. The criticism of getting dishes from the Inner Critic causes one to feel worse and have less desire to adjust. If it's so frustrating to our accumulated experience trying to improve our actions, we stop working. Health psychologists refer to the "abstinence violation effect" spiral of failure-shame-avoidance, which results from violating rigid rules.

Health Happens "In the Middle"

It's unusual that our days go exactly as expected—at work, at home, and anywhere in between. Our children get sick; we get sick; we get stuck in the traffic; we get bad news about the wellbeing of a friend; our supervisor adds a job to our overflowing plate.

Not only is the diet mentality detrimental to weight loss and physical wellbeing; it also runs counter to emotional health. The word cognitive rigidity is used by psychologists to describe thought patterns which are so entrenched that people have difficulty thinking flexibly. Humans are not robots. It's natural to have a hard time implementing a strict plan—whether it's a diet, a "detox," or an effort to give up sugar in cold-turkey. In an ever-changing environment, versatility is key to maintaining healthy eating habits.

The entire notion of versatility is frightening for many people who have struggled with their eating habits, bringing to mind an "everything goes" mindset that can do nothing but curb their unhealthy habits. And that preoccupation is correct. We don't say "anything goes." Having plenty of freedom but no expectations or guidance can leave us wandering in our attempts to make changes—we don't even know where to begin. How then, without being locked into a fixed program, can you make changes?

Behavior-changing progress is most successful when individuals are "in the middle" and not at the extremes. It is crucial to have goals and expectations. However, there is still enough flexibility to allow you to adjust to changing circumstances—including getting off track—to improve your eating habits and continue those changes. It runs counter to the mindset of the diet, and contrary to "everything goes "—and is sustainable.

Get Moving Mindfully

Like healthy food, physical activity (and its lack) plays a significant role in our general wellbeing, our risk of illness, our mental health and happiness, and our weight, of course. But as with food, trends are troubling over the last fifty years, with more and more people living sedentary lives. The numbers are different, but they're grim. Surveys show that just 20 per cent of American adults say they follow the fitness requirements for exercise and strength training, according to the Centers for Disease Control, but the truth could be much worse. Researchers at the National Cancer Institute, who used motion sensors to monitor people more accurately, found that only 5% had at least 30 minutes of moderate-intensity exercise most days of the week.

In January, new participants who plan to work out are filling the gym every day. In the short term, this method can be very motivating but is generally not sustainable. Once again, it's the power-through-it approach, based on external motivation and punishment/reward (think of "no pain, no benefit" and the glistening, unattainable bodies on show in running-shoe ads). To others, starting is too daunting, while many others start and then fizzle out. And some people are overdoing exercise, which can be as harmful as underdoing it. Both of these trends are indicators of shifting outward-in approach.

There is a safe, middle way that begins with yourself tuning in. The why of exercise, as with food, tells them how. Tell yourself,

"What motivates me to exercise? Who do I do this for? "May provide significant detail. For example, you might realize you've been jogging to keep up with (and maybe impress) your athletic sister-in-law, but you don't enjoy it—and what you love is dancing. What if you viewed physical activity as an opportunity to help your overall wellbeing? What if you gain strength, bring joy and fun, and feel confident and competent, instead of concentrating on a specific target (losing a certain amount of weight or fitting into a certain dress), or seeing exercise as something you "should" do? What if you just did it for yourself?

Instead of concentrating on the result, you should focus on the process—miles jogged, pounds lost, calories burned. That means adapting to the way your body feels before, during, and after exercise. That lets you stay versatile. If you know that when swimming your shoulder gets stiff, you should stop before it is an injury—and maybe change your routine to include other activities as well. It helps to differ between a few events for most people, both to avoid damage and to keep off boredom. If you're feeling resistant to the thought of exercise, consider why you're exercising—what you want in the long run. Rather than telling yourself, "Do I feel like doing some exercise?" Mind why this is important to you.

When done in a safe, conscientious way, exercise for a simple purpose is a positive feedback loop: it feels fantastic! And though when you're exercising you feel any pain or exhaustion, you'll experience the benefits shortly after. In fact, with exercise, sometimes the effects are felt faster than with changes in the diet. Our bodies and brains—all from our blood vessels and mitochondria to the feel-good neurotransmitters in our mind—function better when we frequently travel about. It's vital for self-care and overall wellbeing to find your way to the right routine—not too little, not too much, and something you enjoy.

Chapter 32: Guide to Helping Move Forward

Now that you have learned all the components to changing your life for the better when it comes to emotional eating, I am going to leave you with some tips to make sure that you can stay on track and achieve your goals. One of the keys to this that I want to begin with is going into it intending to combine everything you have learned and want to accomplish into one new lifestyle for yourself. This will include your new meal plans, your new snack options, and choices, your continued work on your relationship with food and with yourself, as well as regular exercise. As you begin, it will be difficult, but ease your way into it. And once these all become habits, you won't even notice that you are doing them anymore, and they will become second nature. Anything can become a habit if we practice it for long enough, and these lifestyle changes are no different.

What to Do When It Becomes Difficult

It is inevitable when trying to accomplish something as big as making a change to something that is ingrained in your life-like eating, that it will become difficult at some points along the way. This part will look at what we can do when it becomes painful.

The first thing that you should do is expect it to become difficult at some point. Going into this journey, hoping that it will be a breeze, will only leave you feeling like you have done something wrong when a hard day or a tough week surprises you if you go into this if the mindset that it will become difficult at least a few times, will prevent this from surprising you when it happens and will allow you to appropriately deal with it instead of wondering what you did you cause it.

When it becomes difficult, and you don't know what to eat, you are in a rush, and you have no groceries left, the first thing you want to do is take a deep breath. Then remind yourself why you started in the very first place. Think back on your old ways and how they made you feel. Think of where you are now and praise yourself for what you have accomplished so far, no matter how small. Then, go to the fridge and eat one of the lunches you had intended to take for work tomorrow. By tomorrow, you will likely be having a better day and will have regrouped with your old willpower restored, which will allow you to make a right and healthy decision for your lunch.

Don't get discouraged when something arises that challenges you on your journey. Take it as it comes and tell yourself that this is just what happens in life. Nothing comes without challenges. If something comes up that causes you to slip up and eat something that you would otherwise have chosen not to, don't beat yourself up; just continue with your plan and continue as you would have at the next meal.

Motivation Tips

When you lack motivation, it will help to write about this in your workbook. Sometimes when things become a habit, we forget that they didn't use to be. Think about some of the things that are habits of yours now that were not habits of yours a year ago. This will remind you of what you can accomplish.

Reach out to someone who is supporting you that can provide you with some words of encouragement. This could be anyone who you trust and who you know has your best interests at heart. They will be able to give you some words to motivate you and keep you on track.

Look to support centers online for people recovering from emotional eating or other food-related issues. This can help you to feel that you are not alone and that many other people are facing similar challenges. This will motivate you to keep pushing.

How to Work on Willpower

Willpower is hard to pinpoint, but that is somewhere within all of us. We have to find it somewhere within, and it is there! Think of someone or some people who you think to demonstrate great willpower. Ask yourself what about them shows this. Ask yourself how you think they do this (don't reply with "they just have it"). Ask yourself what other qualities they possess that you admire. Ask yourself if you can pull those same qualities from within yourself. Thinking in this way and trying to emulate a person you admire, and respect will help you to know precisely how willpower looks to you and how willpower displays itself in a person. Having something more concrete to work towards or to reference will help you to find the willpower that is within you.

How to Stick to the Diet

The key to sticking to the diet is one word: preparation. Being prepared for anything will ensure that you won't be able to give yourself any excuse to fall off of the diet. For example, doing all the following:

· Meal prep your lunches.

· Find a place to buy a healthy lunch near your work or school, just in case you forget your lunch one day.

· Prepare a menu for your dinners for the week each weekend.

· Don't buy the snacks that you would usually crave at the grocery store.

· Grocery shop with a specific list and when you are not hungry.

· If you are going out socially, pre-plan what you will order and the number and type of drinks you will have. Then stick to this.

Doing all the above things will make it almost impossible to not stick to the diet. Because everything will be prepared for you already, all you have to do is move the fork to your mouth at every meal, and the diet is stuck to!

How to Reward Yourself as You Hit Milestones

Rewarding yourself is vital as you make your way through this challenging journey. When you hit milestones like one month on the diet or one month without giving in to a craving, then you will keep yourself motivated because you will be working toward your next milestone and, therefore, your next reward each day. Leave enough space between rewards; otherwise, they won't feel as unique. Reward yourself once per month at first and then once every few months as you get more used to everything. You can reward yourself by allowing yourself to buy a medium popcorn at the movie theatre after you have exercised three times a week for a month, for example.

Plan your rewards and write them down on a calendar so that if you are feeling a lack of motivation, you will be able to look at the visual and see how close you are to achieving that goal and that reward. We as creatures love to be rewarded and love to accomplish goals and so giving yourself these options will help you to achieve them.

Conclusion

Let's look back at our progress and then paying it forward to others. Continue eating better all day. You'll feel better, look better, achieve your goals, and have a better quality of life. Assuming you've read and understood all the content here, chances are that you've realized your habits and applying core solutions to overcoming obstacles while holding yourself accountable, you have Paid attention to yourself, your purpose, unique talents, and dreams. By automating your food and water, cutting out unhealthy sugar, alcohol and white carbs, adding protein, Greek yogurt or other probiotics, produce and healthy fats.

Choose to continue with the same eating habit all your life. Focus on a healthy weight; stay with silence. Visualize your step and take steps that are going to get you to where you want to be. If you destabilize procrastination, stress and comfort zone, you will go farther at a fast pace. Organize your kitchen and automate your food. Be a reader; Read positive affirmations aloud every day. Pursue your goals, including your fitness and health goals that will utilize your talents and passions and keep you on the healthy-fit journey. Rest on weekends and follow the process again.

Focus on your activities, journalize your progress, thoughts, and move on. Record your success, nature; they will guide you in thinking and solving stress, among other problems. You will make not only an impact on yourself but also the people around you. Make use of productivity apps on the internet to guide you through.

While writing your journal, consider how you've grown physically, mentally, spiritually, and emotionally or socially. Think about how one area has positively affected other areas. If some things haven't worked out for you, spend some time forgiving other people, forgiving yourself so you can move on. Giving makes living worthwhile.

Albert Einstein believed that a life shared with others is worthy. We have people out there who need you, remember not to hoard your successes. Share your success. Share your new-found recipes, your attitude, and your habits. Share what you have learned with others. In all your undertakings, know that you can't change other people but yourself, therefore, be mindful. Reflect on your changes and put yourself on the back today and every day. Be grateful and live your life as a champion.

Make it a reality on your mind, the fact that the journey to a healthy life and weight loss is long and has many challenges. Pieces of Stuff we consider more important in life require our full cooperation towards them. Just because you are facing problems in your Wight loss journey, it does not mean that you should stop, instead show and prove the whole world how good your ability to handle constant challenges is—training your brain to know that eating healthy food together with functional exercises can work miracles. Make it your choice and not something you are forced to do by a third party. Always tell yourself that weight loss is a long process and not an event. Take every day of your days to celebrate your achievements because these achievements are what piles up to a massive victory. Make a list of stuff you would like to change when you get healthy they may be Small size-clothes, being able to accumulate enough energy, participating in your most loved sports you have been admiring for a more extended period, feeling self-assured. Make these tips your number one source of empowerment; you will end up completing your 30 days even without noticing.

You have made it, or you are about to make it. The journey has been unbelievable. And by now, you must be having a story to tell. Concentrate on finishing strongly. Keep up the excellent eating design you have adopted. Remember, you are not working on temporary changes but long-term goals. Therefore, lifestyle changes should not be stopped when the weight is lost. Remind yourself always of essential habits that are easier to follow daily. They include trusting yourself and the process by acknowledging that the real change lies in your hands. Stop complacency, arise, and walk around for at least thirty minutes away. Your breakfast is the most important meal you deserve. Eat your breakfast like a queen. For each diet, you take, add a few proteins and natural fats. Let hunger not kill you, eat more, but just what is recommended, bring snacks and other meals 3 or 5 times a day. Have more veggies and fruits like 5-6 rounds in 24 hours. Almost 90% of Americans do not receive enough vegetables and fruits to their satisfaction. Remember, Apple will not make you grow fat. Substitute salt. You will be shocked by the sweet taste of food once you stop consuming salt. Regain your original feeling, you will differentiate natural flavorings from artificial flavors. Just brainstorm how those older adults managed to eat their food without salt or modern-day characters. Characters are not suitable for your health. Drink a lot of water in a day. Let water be your number one drink. Avoid soft drinks and other energy drinks, and they are slowly killing you. Drink a lot of water in the morning after getting out of your bed. Your body will be fresh from morning to evening. Have a journal and be realistic with it. Take charge of what you write and be responsible.

Rapid Weight Loss
Hypnosis and Meditation

Table of Contents

Introduction

"I know I can do anything I set my mind to because I am strong and confident." Affirmations like this one are intended to lift a person's spirits when they are feeling low or anxious. Affirmations can be about anything and are relatively easy to think of so long as they are positive. When you say this statement to yourself, "I am perfect just the way that I am," you don't have to necessarily believe it, but they are vital for personal growth. It has been proven that people who tell themselves at least one good thing (whether they believed that statement or not) have less stressful days and are generally happier than those who don't. Positive reinforcement is absolutely essential for the purpose of losing weight because those who struggle with their weight usually feel overwhelmed, stressed, depressed, or believe that they are unworthy. With this type of mindset, it's no wonder you're unhappy with your weight. There are so many things in life that can bring you down, but your own bodyweight doesn't need to be one of them.

When people are upset, they will oftentimes either starve themselves or eat comfort food to make them feel better. You probably got interested in this because you realized that you're in an unhealthy cycle. First, you may have had something happen to you during the day that has stressed you out, which you will then ruminate and obsess over how ugly you think you are. Negative thoughts lead to poor self-image and low self-esteem, which can make anyone depressed or angry. So, the next (unhealthy) step is usually grabbing a slice of cake, a bag of chips, a chocolate brownie, or any other junk food to make you feel better. While you're eating it, you feel better, but then afterward, you realize you may have gone too far and start to feel ashamed, embarrassed, or even guilty. These feelings then trigger another emotional response, which stresses you out, and here we are back at the beginning again. It is a vicious, unending circle.

This will help you control your mindset by getting you to feel uplifted and confident about developing positive habits to healthy eating and regular exercise. Don't think that meditation alone will decrease your weight, because there are other things that you can do to continue taking the pounds off to reach your ideal body weight. However, reading about meditation, affirmations, and hypnosis will help you become motivated to lose the pounds as if they were never a problem in the first place. The core issue here is that your brain is stuck in this negative cycle, which is one of the leading causes of binge eating and automatic eating. Have you ever noticed that when you eat a bunch of carbs and processed foods, you feel sluggish and have deficient energy? That's because those foods have nothing good in them. The idea of hypnosis is to bring you to a subconscious state and trick your mind, so you don't feel a certain way, and the affirmations are to help build your self-esteem, so you feel like getting up and walking or going for a run, maybe you'll be inspired to grab a gym membership. Meditation is used to help you relax and train your mind not to think negatively, so you can better focus on your goals ahead.

Throughout the meditations here, I promise that you will be well on your way to success and become motivated to reach your desired body weight. Remember, you don't have to be perfect to complete your goals; as long as you are always trying, you will always succeed. Throughout this topic, make sure that you are either lying flat on a comfortable surface or sitting naturally in a comfortable chair. Also try to avoid stressful environments, such as a workspace or office, a place with noisy pets, children, or other people in general. The goal before starting each exercise is to have your mind clear so that these exercises can work. Bring only positive energy into your being and listen carefully to the meditations.

Chapter 1: What is Hypnosis for Weight Loss?

Hypnosis is a great way to help those in need of weight loss. There are various reasons a person may be overweight. Some may range from behavioral issues or underlying conditions that will require to be addressed to lose weight successfully. After losing weight, a person needs to maintain it.

Does Hypnosis Accelerate Your Weight Loss?

Those that have utilized entrancing to help in weight reduction have revealed incredible enhancements at the speed in which they had the option to shed the pounds. Here, we will talk about how this happens, utilizing suggestions from those that have attempted and succeeded.

Spellbinding is an instrument utilized by certain advisors to help individuals accomplish total unwinding. Specialists believe that the cognizant and oblivious personality can concentrate and concentrate on verbal reiteration and mental imaging during a session. As an outcome, the psyche winds up open to recommendations and open to modifying in conduct, emotions, and practices.

Since the 1700s, types of this elective treatment have been utilized to help people from bed-wetting to nail-gnawing to smoking with anything. Spellbinding examination, as we will research in this paper, has likewise demonstrated some guarantee to treat corpulence.

Mesmerizing might be progressively productive for people who need to get in shape than eating regimen and exercise alone. The idea is that to change practices like gorging; the psyche can be influenced. Be that as it may, it is as yet being tackled decisively how effective it tends to be.

What's in store from hypnotherapy

By clarifying how mesmerizing functions, your specialist will most likely begin your session during the hypnotherapy. At that point, they will go past your private goals. Your specialist can begin talking in an unwinding, delicate tone from that point to help you unwind and make a suspicion that all is well and good.

When you have arrived at an increasingly open perspective, your advisor may propose techniques to help adjust eating or practicing rehearses or different strategies to accomplish your destinations of weight reduction.

With this point, certain words or redundancy of specific sentences can help. Your specialist may likewise help you to envision yourself by trading striking mental symbolism to accomplish targets.

Your advisor will help you escape trance and back to your beginning state to close the session. The term of the mesmerizing session and the total measure of sessions you may need will depend on your targets. In as few as one to three gatherings, a few people may see results.

Types of Hypnotherapy

Different sorts of hypnotherapy exist. For propensities, for example, smoking, nail-gnawing, and dietary issues, recommended treatment is all the more as often as possible utilized.

Together with different meds, for example, healthful guidance or CBT, your specialist may likewise utilize hypnotherapy.

Hypnotherapy expenses change depending on where you live and the specialist you pick. Think about calling forward to talk about choices for estimating or sliding scale.

Your protection business can cover somewhere in the range of 50 and 80% of affirmed experts ' treatment. Call for more data about your inclusion once more.

You can find authorized specialists by mentioning a referral from your essential doctor or via looking through the suppliers ' database of the American Society for Clinical Hypnosis.

Points of interest for Hypnotherapy

Studies demonstrate that a few people might be increasingly responsive and, in this way, bound to profit by the effects of entrancing, for example, an individual might be progressively inclined to mesmerizing by certain character qualities, benevolence and transparency.

Research has likewise found that mesmerizing helplessness ascends after age 40, and females are progressively plausible to be open paying little mind to age. Under the direction of an affirmed trance specialist, spellbinding is viewed as a protected practice with not many reactions, for example:

- Headache

- Dizziness

- Drowsiness

- Anxiety trouble

- Fake memory creation

Individuals who are masters in visualizations or daydreams should converse with their primary care physician before psychotherapy is explored. Likewise, affected by drug or liquor, the mental state ought not to be performed on a private person.

Extra weight reduction tips

- Here are a few things you can do at home to enable you to get more fit:

- Move your body on most days of the week. Attempt to get either 150 minutes of moderate action (for example, strolling, water heart stimulating exercise, cultivating) or 75 minutes of progressively lively work out (for example running, swimming, climbing) each week.

- Keep a day by day dinner. Track the amount you eat, when you eat, and if you eat from yearning or not. Doing so can enable you to recognize evolving propensities, for example, fatigue eating.

- Eat vegetables and natural products. Go for five foods grown from the ground servings consistently. To check your craving, you ought to likewise add more fiber to your eating routine—between 25 to 30 grams every day.

- Drink water each day from six to eight glasses. Being hydrated abstains from eating excessively.

- The inclination to skip suppers is safe. Eating throughout the day keeps up your digestion going incredible.

Chapter 2: Heal Your Relationship with Food

A straightforward method to perform this is to keep a food journal and a mood journal. Write down each time you know you've consumed unhealthy foods. Look back later on what feelings make you eat. You'll be able to recognize patterns or beliefs that make you overeat as time goes by. When you know what is causing your emotional eating, you will start working on how to avoid it and find ways to eat healthier.

1. Find other ways to fuel your emotions.

When you can't find another way to deal with your feelings without requiring food, so breaking this practice would be almost impossible. One of the reasons diets fail is that they give rational nutrition recommendations under the premise that lack of awareness is the only thing that stops you from eating properly. That form of suggestion only works if you can control eating habits. It's not enough to recognize your causes and grasp your process to stop emotional eating—you need to find new ways to cope with your emotions. You can call or have a hangout with a friend who makes you feel better when you're depressed or lonely, visit places you like, read an interesting book, watch a comedy show or play with the cat.

2. When cravings arrive, pause.

This might not be as simple as it sounds, because it is all you might think about when the desire for the food hits. You feel right there, and then, the need to feed. Taking at least five minutes before you give up on the craving, this gives you time to think about the wrong decision you're about to make. You can change your mind at that time and make a better choice. Start with 2 minutes if 5 minutes is a lot for you and increasing the time as you get better with it.

3. Learn to embrace good feelings and negative ones.

Emotional eating comes from being unable to cope with the feelings on the brain. Find a friend or therapist who will speak to you about the problems and concerns you have. Being willing to accept negative and good emotions without having to include food would improve change.

4. Commit to healthy lifestyle habits.

Exercise, rest and adequate sleep will make it easier for you to deal with any emotional or physical problem you may experience. Create time for at least five days a week for a 30-minute workout, relax, and sleep 7 to 8 hours a day. It's also essential to surround yourself with caring people who will empower you and help you cope with your issues.

The first thing to keep emotional eating in mind is the addictive effect food has on you. You may encounter cravings that often feel uncontrollable, and you may feel as though you are addicted to food much as a smoker is addicted to smoking. The trick is to properly control your emotions and feelings and train your brain not to respond to stressful or unpleasant feelings by merely having to eat food (your preference brain drug) to calm down.

There are a few other useful methods and approaches that you can use to avoid emotional eating and lose weight, including: abandon the Diet!

Dieting ruins your metabolism, and you can eventually find yourself taking on weight. In reality, dieting will only work in the short run and will lower your fragile self-esteem.

Adjust your way of thinking.

Don't equate to anyone.

When you lose weight, it is crucial not to equate your weight with the importance of those around you. If you're unhappy with your weight, comparing yourself to the skinny girls you see in magazines or on television could prolong your recovery process by adjusting your lifestyle habits with eating, exercise, and mind control; you'll find it much easier to stop emotional eating and lose the weight you want much faster and longer-term.

When you've mastered techniques for managing your eating causes, your emotional food cravings should cease.

In a person who is in control of their emotions and has more constructive ways of coping with negative feelings, emotional eating cannot thrive, it is unlikely. You can eat intuitively before you know it and be free from raw food and excess body fat for good.

Over-food is still not given the due treatment it deserves. It is always seen as not a real issue and to be laughing at something.

That view is entirely false because it is a horrific illness that needs urgent care. The positive news is that taking action to help yourself avoid emotional eating forever is easy to do. I say that because I did it myself.

Stage # 1-Identifying the causes.

For each person, emotional eating is caused differently. Some people get the cravings when stressed out, and some when depressed or bored. You have to think a bit to figure out what your emotional causes are. When you know what they are, you will be given early notice when the desire to eat comes upon you.

Step # 2-Eliminating Temptation.

The one thing many people don't know about emotional eating is that often the craving is for one particular food. It is mostly ice-cream or candy for kids. Usually, for people, it's pizza. If you couldn't satisfy this temptation, that's not going to bother you as much. Clear out any of these temptations from your house. Throw out any nearby pizza delivery places. Once you know your tempters, get rid of them and make overeating hard for you.

Step # 3-The link breaks.

When the impulse hits, it's intense and instant. You are now feeling like eating. Good! You need to break this immediate bond by giving yourself some time between the desire and the eating to avoid this.

• Call a friend

• Count to 60

• Write down what you feel

• Do some exercises

• Go outside for a walk

• Take a shower.

Whatever you can do to let the urge subside do wonder. Take these three steps, and you'll be doing them easier early and conquer emotional eating for good.

Would you like to learn the best ideas on how emotional eating stops working? It's emotional eating that satisfies your sensitive appetite. It has nothing to do with your kitchen, but in your mind lies the issue. What are the most potent methods to overcome the emotional eating temptation? Make a list to relieve your cravings for food.

Prepare for future emotional eating issues. Draw a piece of paper and a pencil over the weekend and take a route about your activities in the days ahead. Your map will show the stops you intend to make and potential detours. Choose an icon that reflects emotional eating. Place the image over an occurrence or activity that could cause your cravings for food, like an early lunch with your in-laws. Prepare ahead for that case. Look for the restaurant menu online so you can order something delicious but still good.

Clear the fears inside out. It helps if you take a deep breath, anytime you are nervous. Another thing you should do is to do a visual trick to detoxify yourself from the stress. Breathe in deeply and imagine a squeegee put near your head (that piece of cloth you use to clean your window or windshield). Breathe out slowly, and believe the squeegee is wiping clean your heart. With it taking away all the worries. Do this quad.

Self-talk as if you're royalty. Usually, self-criticism goes to emotional eating. Toxic words you say to yourself, such as "I'm such a loser" or "I can't seem to be doing anything right", force you to drive to the closest. Don't be misled even though these claims are brief. Such feelings are like acid rain, which is slowly eroding your wellbeing. The next time you're caught telling yourself these negative words, counteracting by moving to a third-person perspective. In moments when you think "I'm such a mess", then remind yourself that "Janice is such a mess, but Janice will do what it takes to make it work out and make herself happy". This approach will help you out of the negative self-talk loop and give you some perspective. Pull up and be positive, and you'll have the strength to avoid emotional eating.

How can hypnosis aid with weight loss keep you stuck in a vicious cycle?

Hypnotherapy is aimed at improving your eating habits and increased levels of trust and encouragement to help you achieve success. There are six steps to the Goldcrest Hypnotherapy Weight Loss plan to be effective in losing weight for good:

1. Establish ATTITUDE ON RIGHT.

To lose weight, you must be inspired, determined and focused. Hypnotherapy can help you to be optimistic and to trust that you will lose weight and lead a healthier life. It should reframe your thoughts and empower you to take full responsibility for handling your pressure. Part of the hypnotherapy is to concentrate on the habits of self-defeating thinking that might have caused you to give up in the past.

2. No. Establish Habits, HEALTHY EATING.

If your mentality is right and fired up, I'll help you let go of the unhealthy eating habits and motivate you to lose weight by adopting healthy eating habits. The purpose is to help you regain control over food and increase your desire to lead a healthy life, including increased exercise wherever possible. The counselling should involve recognizing patterns of eating and seeking ways to improve eating habits. I'm going to help you build an eating plan that follows 80-20 law. You'll eat 80% of the time comfortably and have a bit of what you'd like for the remaining 20%.

3. Think about it. SET GOALS Low.

You may want to be the same size that you were when you were at college. But that could mean a five stone loss. Don't set such a big target for yourself. Divide the broad goal into smaller objectives. Set yourself 5 per cent or 10 per cent lower, more achievable targets and allow yourself a much longer timeline to accomplish it.

Giving yourself a bit of flexibility is also necessary. Your weight-loss journey will have ups and downs. It's essential your weight loss program is not static but flexible; otherwise, it won't feel like it suits into your life.

4. No. SET Target SPECIFIC.

Should not set common targets such as: "I have to consume less food," or "I have to do more".

Instead, set specific short-term goals such as: "I'm going to take a healthy lunch to work every day instead of going to a fast-food restaurant" or "I'm going to go on a Monday and Wednesday night after work every week for a 30-minute walk with my friend".

5. EAT BREAKFAST ALL TODAY.

Most people miss breakfast for being too busy or not hungry. Eat slow foods which release energy, such as oats, that will keep you going until lunch.

Set your alarm ahead of time. Make sure you go to bed 15 minutes sooner, so you don't cut down on your overall sleep.

Chapter 3: Relaxation to Promote Physical Healing

Since we have seen that emotions are the first obstacle to a healthy and correct relationship with food, we are going to look specifically at the most suitable techniques to appease them. Not only that, but these techniques are also very important to make hypnosis deeply effective in order to achieve the desired goals.

This is all about hypnosis. In particular, the one for virtual gastric banding. But in addition to hypnosis, it is worth spending a few words on autogenic training. You will thus have a technique that you can use anywhere without external aids and which can also increase the effectiveness of hypnosis. That will lead to greater awareness of the mind-body relationship.

In fact, autogenic training is one of the techniques of self-hypnosis. What does self-hypnosis mean? As the word suggests, it is a form of self-induced hypnosis. Beyond the various techniques available, all have the objective of concentrating a single thought object. To say it seems easy, but it is incredible how in reality our mind is constantly distracted and even overlaps distant thoughts between them. This leads to emotional tension with repercussions in everyday life.

Other self-hypnosis techniques that we will not deal with in-depth include Benson's and Erickson's.

Benson's is inspired by oriental transcendental meditation. it is based on the constant repetition of a concept in order to favor a great concentration. Specifically, he recommends repeating the word that evokes the concept several times. It is the easiest and fastest technique ever. It really takes 10-15 minutes a day. Just because it's so simple doesn't mean it's not effective. And you will also need to familiarize yourself with it, especially for those who are beginners with self-hypnosis. In fact, this could be the first technique to try right away to approach this type of practice.

You sit with your eyes closed in a quiet room and focus on breathing and relax the muscles. Therefore, you need to think about the object of meditation continually. If your thought turns away, bring it back to the object. To be sure to practice this self-hypnosis at least 10 minutes, just set a timer.

Erickson's is apparently more complex. The first step involves creating a new self-image that you would like to achieve. So, we start from something we don't like about ourselves and mentally create a positive image that we would like to create.

In our specific case, we could start from the idea of us being overweight and transform that idea into an image of us in perfect shape, satisfied with ourselves in front of the mirror.

Then we focus on three objects around the subject then three noises and finally three sensations. It takes little time to concentrate on these things. Gradually decrease this number. Therefore 2 objects, 2 noises and 2 sensations. Better if the objects are small and bright and unusual sensations, which are hardly paid attention. For example, the feeling of the shirt that we wear in contact with our skin. You get to one and then you leave your mind wandering. We take the negative image we have and calmly transform it mentally into the positive one. At the end of this practice you will feel great energy and motivation.

Autogenic Training

Autogenic training is a highly effective self-induced relaxation technique without external help. It is called "training" because it includes a series of exercises that allow the gradual and passive acquisition of changes in muscle tone, vascular function, cardiac and pulmonary activity, neuro-vegetative balance, and state of consciousness. But do not be frightened by this word. His exercises do not require a theoretical preparation nor a radical modification of one's habits. Practicing this activity always allows you to live a profound and repeatable experience.

Autogenic means "self-generating", unlike hypnosis and self-hypnosis which are actively induced by an operator or the person himself.

The goal is to achieve inner harmony so that we can best face the difficulties of everyday life. It is a complementary tool for hypnosis. The two activities are intertwined. Practicing both allows a better overall experience. In fact, hypnosis helps well to act directly on the subconscious. But for hypnosis to be effective, it is necessary to have already prepared an inner calm such that there is no resistance to the instructions given by the hypnotherapist. The origins of autogenic training are rooted in the activity of hypnosis. In the latter, there is an exclusive relationship between hypnotist and hypnotized. Those who are hypnotized must, therefore, be in a state of maximum receptivity to be able to reach a state of constructive passivity in order to create the ideal relationship with the hypnotists.

Those who approach autogenic training and have already undergone hypnosis sessions can deduce the main training guidelines from the principles of hypnosis. The difference is that you become your own hypnotist. You must, therefore, assume an attitude of receptive availability towards you. Such activity also allows a higher spiritual introspection, feeling masters of one's emotional state. This undoubtedly brings countless advantages in everyday life.

So, I usually suggest everyone try a hypnosis session and then do a few days of autogenic training before they start using hypnosis again daily. It is the easiest way to approach the relaxation techniques on your own and start to become familiar with the psycho-physical sensations given by these practices. Mine is a spontaneous suggestion. If you have tried meditation and relaxation techniques in the past, you can also go directly into guided hypnosis. In any case, autogenic training can be useful regardless of the level of familiarity with these practices. If you have little time in your days, it makes no sense to put so much meat on the fire. Let us remember that they are still relaxation techniques if we see them too much as "training" we could associate obligations and bad emotions that go against the principle of maximum relaxation. So, I'm not saying do autogenic training and hypnosis every day, 10 push-ups, crunches and maybe yoga and then you will be relaxed and at peace with your body. This approach is not good. It is about finding your balance and harmony in a practice that must be pleasant and deliberate.

Basic Autogenic Training Exercises

The basic exercises of the A.T. are classically divided into 6 exercises of which 2 fundamental and 4 complementary. Before the 6 exercises, you practice an induction to calm and relaxation, while at the end a recovery and then awakening.

These exercises are considered as consecutive phases to be carried out in each session. It is not mandatory to carry out all the steps together. Especially initially, each exercise will have to be understood individually. But if you intend to stop, for example, in the fourth exercise, and not do all of them, you will necessarily have to do the other 3 exercises in the same session first. The duration of the session remains unchanged, however, because when you add exercises you will make each phase last less. You will add the exercise when you feel you have learned the preceding one.

First Exercise - "The heaviness." It's a very useful exercise to overcome psychophysical problems related to muscular tensions that derive from emotional tensions.

Second Exercise - "The heat." It serves to relieve circulatory problems, in all cases where there is a problem of reduced blood flow to the extremities.

Third Exercise - "The heart." It is a highly suggestive exercise that allows you to regain contact with that part of the body that we traditionally deal with emotions.

Fourth Exercise - "The breath." It produces a better oxygenation of the blood and organs.

Fifth Exercise: - The solar plexus. It helps a lot of those who suffer from digestive problems.

Sixth Exercise - The Fresh Forehead. Produces a brain constriction vessel that can be especially useful to reduce headaches, especially if linked to physical or mental overload.

Recommended positions.

The following positions are suitable for both autogenic training and hypnosis and relaxation techniques in general. I suggest initially to use the lying down position and to use it in hypnosis for virtual gastric bandaging to simulate the position on the surgical couch.

Lying Down.

This position, at least at the beginning, is the most used for its comfort. You lie on your back (face up) and your legs slightly apart with your toes out. The arms are slightly detached from the torso and are slightly bent. The fingers are detached from each other and slightly arched.

On the Armchair

You sit with a chair attached to the wall. Your back is firmly against the backrest and your head rests against the wall. You can place a cushion between your head and the wall.

Alternatively, you can use a high chair to rest your head-on. Legs should be flexed at 90 degrees with the feet firmly resting on them. The tips of the feet should be placed on the outside. The arms should be resting on the supports (where present) or on the thighs.

If there are supports, the hands should be left dangling.

If they are not present, the hands are resting on the legs and the fingers are separate.

Other suggestions

To achieve the best results, the environment must be quiet, the phone and any form of technological distraction must be disconnected beforehand. In the room there must be an incredibly soft light with a constant temperature that allows neither hot nor cold. The environmental conditions, in fact, influence our mood, and the acquisition of a correct position guarantees an objective relaxation of all the muscles.

It is advisable not to wear clothes that tighten or bother you during the exercises: for this purpose, also remove the watch and glasses and loosen the belt.

It goes without saying that constancy is especially important for achieving a psychic balance. It only takes 10 minutes a day but a real reluctance is to be taken into consideration. Before doing this practice, you really need to give yourself some time. It must be a deliberate practice. This is one of the reasons why it is not advisable to practice it in small time gaps between commitments, but rather in dedicated time slots.

Also, it is advisable not to practice the exercises immediately after lunch to avoid sleep. At the end of each workout, perform awakening exercises except for the evening just before going to sleep. At first, checking the relaxation of the various parts of the body will require some reflection. But over time and practice, everything will become more instinctive. Do not expect great results in the first days of practice, do not abandon the practice immediately because like anything else, you cannot expect to know how to do it immediately.

One last tip is to not be too picky when it comes to checking the position to take. In fact, the indications provided are broad, it is not necessary to interpret them rigidly. It must be as natural as possible, so look for what makes you feel better.

Chapter 4: The Power of Guided Meditation

When you want to find ways to meditate calmly, you can try your hand at some other techniques that are designed to help you focus and settle your thoughts. One of the best methods to clear your head is to use your mantras or your affirmations in mantra meditation.

Find a comfortable place to sit and rest yourself cross-legged with your hands on your knees. Try to keep your spine straight, as slumping is a posture of defeat, and you want to keep an aura of confidence. Choose a mantra to recite in your head or try to recite your affirmation if it's not too long.

Close your eyes and try to imagine a candle burning. Focus on the flame as you slowly inhale and exhale. Basic yoga breathing works well for this meditation method. As you inhale, keep your mind's eye on the flame. As you exhale, think about your mantra, reciting it in your head or aloud. You can also use your goals or your milestones as your recitation. For example, if you are nearing a landmark in your weight loss plan, try using it during your meditation, like this:

Inhale, focused on the flame…

Exhale, say, "I'll hit my ten-pound mark this week."

Continue this exercise until you find your concentration flagging. You may need to start slow, working in five-minute increments, until you can meditate for a longer, more effective period. Every little bit counts when it comes to mantra meditation.

Another effective meditation for focus is a practice known as gazing. This technique is performed by choosing an object to study carefully and giving it your full attention until it's the only thing you are thinking about. Find your object and either hold it if it's small enough or sit near it if it's too large to hold. Trinkets like jewelry work for this meditation, as do simple pieces of artwork or an interesting article of clothing like a patterned scarf.

Sitting comfortably, use yoga breathing to calm yourself down, then begin to look at your object. You want to observe all its obvious qualities, beginning with things like color and shape. Continue your observations, asking yourself, what does it feel like? Is it light or heavy? Take in all the physical properties of your chosen object. Think about the texture of the materials and the way the light reflects off of it. You want the only thing in the world to be the object in your gaze. Try not to look away; breaking your gaze will break the meditation. When you can no longer find anything new to observe about the object, close your eyes, and describe it to yourself. When you've finished, take a few deep breaths and open your eyes.

The idea behind gazing is to be able to concentrate all your energy on one goal, to keep your eyes on the prize literally. When you can use gazing as an effective meditation, you will learn to build stamina and focus, which will help you further your weight loss goals, and in fact, any other goals you should choose to set for yourself.

Another great way to meditate quietly is to make a recording and play it back to yourself while you focus on your own words. Self-guided meditation is a wonderful way to lift yourself and remind yourself of your accomplishments thus far. You can use the voice recorder or video recorder application on your phone or a small digital recorder like a reporter might use for interviews. It takes little work, but write yourself a short script or some notes, and make a positive soundtrack for yourself.

You can record yourself talking over a backdrop of soothing music, with breaks in between so the tune can relax you as well. Aim for recording time of five to ten minutes, even if you only speak for a few minutes, and you edit a loop. Read your affirmation to yourself, calmly recite your mantras, or just give yourself a low-key pep talk. When it's time to meditate, find a comfy place to sit, take a few deep breaths, pop in your earphones, and press play. Focus on your own words lifting you to your next goal; it will do you a world of good as you move to your next milestone.

With all these meditation techniques to choose from, you may be thinking we're running out of methods to talk about, but we haven't even gotten to mindfulness yet! Meditation and mindfulness aren't the same, but they are allies to each other and you as you seek to lose weight and achieve a healthier lifestyle. Let's keep moving and see what mindfulness can do for you.

Chapter 5: Body Image Relaxation

From the preceding part, you have got the meditation exercises that you can use to help you move in the right direction when it comes to your weight loss goal. Maybe you have always wanted to do this, and in the past, you have tried to do some of the exercises like the centering ones such as Circle of Light, contemplation, or breathe counting. You have also chosen the most relevant program for weight control, like doing the Where Am I hungry? In addition, Petal Lotus meditations, and you are doing the balance scale meditation. The meditations are helping you, and now you can avoid opening the fridge to quench your urge since you are doing one of the meditations you have already chosen.

This is a wonderful program, and it can help you to achieve your goals and maintain the right weight for your body. Nevertheless, the truth is that you do not need this only because you need preparedness for some moments when you find that you are stressed up, and the way things are difficult there is the possibility of being pushed to the wall until you break your program and even your diet. This is the time when you find yourself deciding to eat when you do not necessarily need food because you are looking for comfort, and you want to soothe your body. For example, when you receive that one call and get to know that one of your plans that you have been planning carefully cannot happen, or you know that something important you depend on will not be functioning anymore and many other difficult issues that may surround you at different moments.

Are you able to handle and deal with the kind of stress that builds up during these moments? How do you do when you find yourself that you are facing the type of stress that makes you feel so hungry such that you feel like you have been starving for many days. Many people forget about the meditation program when this happens, and they find themselves the only thing they can do is to start eating whatever they can find in their environment because all they want is to feel the comfort. They result in emotional eating, and without realizing, they eventually find that they have gained the weight they tried to reduce, and all the work they did is gone. While these meditation exercises can help you to achieve your weight goals, there are these special moments when you find

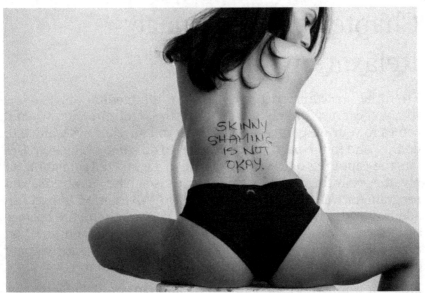

that pressure has built up so much. The following thing that will happen to you is that you may result in your old eating habits and start eating food that is not needed in your body biologically.

This is one of the worst situations that can happen because when you result in the bad old habits of eating, you will gain this unwanted food, and the best thing you can do at the moment is know how you can control this situation. In the following part, we will look at some of the best meditations that you can use to help you to handle these difficult times so that you are not disrupted from doing your meditations on a daily basis. These meditations are necessary to ensure as other people have done before, you do not fall into the trap of staying away from your meditation exercises and going back to your old eating habits, which makes you gain weight that is not necessary for your body. However, you need to understand that the meditations in these parts should be added to the already meditations that you are using and not substituted.

Life will not always be rosy, and you can be sure that at some point, you will find yourself in a difficult situation such that you have a lot of emotional eating. Some people try their best to maintain their meditation program, but it comes to a point when they are not able to continue it because of the difficult things they are facing in life. For example, imagine when you lose your job, and you have your family to feed, and you have nothing else you can do at the moment to earn income. This is why the meditation exercises during difficult times are crucial and should be incorporated in your daily meditations for weight loss because they will help you to ensure that you are pushing. Time does not come when you find that you are not able to do it. When you find yourself facing rough times, you need to practice these meditations around three to four hours and choose the one you feel is the right one for you. When you assume there are difficulties ahead, it is essential since you will be equipped with what you need for the future. When you are prepared for what may happen on your way to your destination, the chances are you will achieve it since you can do away with the obstacles and are now able to move on with your regular program.

As such, you need to take your time to read every meditation in this part and ensure that you practice severally to get everything right since they will help you in your journey to attain the right body weight. Also, as you do the meditations in the following part, make sure that you can make sense out of each. The good thing is that when you maintain your discipline at this time and master everything well, the moment you find that you have hit a tough path, you will be in a position to move on and doing away with emotional eating, which can lead to weight, gain. Remember that there is no certainty in modern life, and even the best plans can fail in the last moment when you had thought that you have almost achieved what you wanted. You cannot predict anything, and there is always pain and difficulty as you live.

Chapter 6: How to Use Meditation and Affirmations to Lose Weight

Your dominant habits, beliefs, and mental attitude (your circumstance) come from thoughts, which is why you need to become aware of them lest you attract unseemly circumstances, habits, and beliefs and therefore an unseemly life that never helps you achieve your full potential of which you know you have a lot of.

The average human has between 6,000-70,000 thoughts per day. Because some of these thoughts are fleeting, what we can only call "musings of the mind," thoughts are not equal. The most powerful thoughts, the ones that can change your life, are those you attach the most emotional power to and think of frequently.

Awareness of thought is a learned habit that asks you to learn how to balance between obsessively monitoring all your thoughts—including fleeting ones that have a minimal effect on your life—and awareness of your most habitual thoughts.

Thought awareness is not obsessing over every thought; it is aware of your habitual thoughts because, as we have said, only the thoughts you repeat and attach emotions to have the ability to change your life.

A large percentage of our thoughts are habitual. Science estimates that because of the vast number of thoughts experienced by the human mind per day, 95-99% of our thoughts and behaviors are automatic.

Because the mind is a professional automation machine—it automates to save brainpower—without awareness of thought, it is possible to create a reality that is vastly different from the one you desire. For instance, if you want a new job or house but your most common thoughts or beliefs towards that undertaking are negative or you consider yourself undeserving of these things, your circumstances will change only after you change your thoughts and, therefore, beliefs and habits.

Habitually embed these affirmations into your subconscious mind and your state of health shall change or improve. Imbedded into

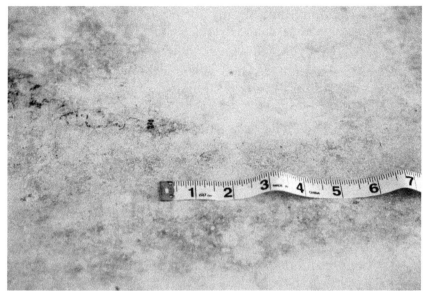

the subconscious mind repeatedly, these affirmations can help you communicate better with your body to heal and achieve overall mental and physical wellbeing.

Remember that the emotions attached to the words are as important as making the thought habitual.

1. "I am healthy."

2. "Every part of my body is in perfect health."

3. "My mind and body are allying that work with me for my overall good."

4. "Universal life force flows through me, healing and nourishing every part of my body, mind, and being."

5. "My body functions well."

6. "The cells in my body work together and quickly to bring about swift healing."

7. "My body and mind are partners that work together to foster my overall wellbeing."

8. "I am a radiant ray of positive energy."

9. "Because I am thought aware, I control my thoughts. I cultivate thoughts of wellbeing, which is why I reap wellbeing in my daily life."

10. "My body and mind are my greatest allies. They easily

communicate with me about what I need to live a life of good health and overall wellbeing."

11. "My health is my greatest source of wealth, which is why I love it and take good care of it through mind and body nutrition (positive thinking, food, exercise and nutrition)."

12. "The connections between my mind and body are clear highways of communication."

13. "I love my body. I always give it what it needs to heal quickly and efficiently."

14. "Through thought awareness, I control my health and wellbeing by ensuring the thoughts most common in my mind are healthy."

15. "Good health is my habit. I nourish and care for my body every minute of every day."

16. "Every day in every way, I am healthier and stronger."

17. "I am in perfect health."

18. "My body knows how to repair and heal itself."

19. "My wellbeing thoughts are healthy. They bloom into my reality as perfect health."

20. "I am grateful for perfect health and overall wellbeing as I work towards fulfilling my greatest potential."

Remember that the emotions you attach to the affirmation matters too. Attach emotions of wellbeing, happiness, good health, and intuition about your life as you pursue your purpose.

Affirmations to Heal Your Body When It Is Sick

To bring about positivity into your mind and body when you are not feeling well, you need to practice loving-kindness affirmations.

Below are some affirmations for that:

21. "I am always kind to myself."

22. "I always treat my body kindly."

23. "When my body gets sick, I treat it with kindness. I give it

everything it needs to heal and recuperate quickly."

24. "I always carry in me and transmit to the universe loving kindness to my body and mind, loved ones, my community, and the world/universe around me."

25. "I transmit a radiant ray of loving-kindness towards my body and mind."

26. "My body has the ability to process and release all emotions that are not beneficial to my health and overall wellbeing."

27. "Because I believe in my body's ability to heal, I deserve to heal."

28. "I believe in my body's ability to heal efficiently."

29. "I am not my circumstances. I love myself despite this illness."

30. "This disease is not who I am. I am healthy, because of which I love myself and always care for my body. I always give it what it needs to heal itself."

31. "I always give my body the rest it needs to heal and recuperate."

32. "I believe I am deserving of healing."

33. "I choose to be positive about my health. I am in alignment with my mind, body, and all their needs."

34. "I think positive thoughts about my health and my body's ability to heal itself."

35. "My body is resilient. It knows it has the ability to fight off any illness that may afflict it."

36. "My body knows what to do to ease stress and overcome all forms of illnesses that hinder my overall wellbeing."

37. "I accept and appreciate my body as it is right now."

38. "My body always does its best to ensure I'm in perfect health."

39. "I show my love and appreciation towards my body by exercising and eating right."

40. "I am a vibrant ray of perfect health and loving-kindness towards myself, others, and the universe at large."

Creating Health or Sickness Affirmations

As you now know, these are but a few health affirmations to get you started. As an earlier part taught, you can easily create your own, customized affirmations following a few rules.

When creating healing affirmations, make a point of using words such as willing, time, choose, allow and other words that show your resolve or decision. The subconscious mind is a slave that lacks the ability to disobey a conscious command. In addition, keep in mind that belief is of utmost importance. If you fail to attach emotions to a healing affirmation (belief is a strong emotion), it will not work. Ensure that at some level, you believe the affirmations.

Another important thing worth mentioning is the need to keep your health affirmations positive and present-oriented. Their phrasing should be present-oriented so that you can experience healing in the present moment.

Positive Thinking Affirmations

A positive mind is a breeding ground for a positive life. In fact, to use affirmations to influence and change any area of your life, you first need to become a positive thinker. Like most things worth pursuing or having, positive thinking is a habit that you can develop by saturating your conscious and subconscious mind with positive words, phrases, and sentences/affirmations.

Below are 20 positivity-inclined affirmations:

41. "I am a positivity magnet."

42. "Positive thoughts saturate my mind."

43. "I attract positivity."

44. "I am not my circumstances; I create my circumstances."

45. "I am healthy, wealthy, happy, and fulfilled."

46. "I believe in my abilities and potentials."

47. "I am strong-willed and resilient."

48. "I am a conqueror."

49. "I spread positivity everywhere I go and to everyone I meet."

50. "I attract into my life positive circumstances and people."

51. "I have the ability to overcome anything that life throws at me."

52. "My mind, body, and spirit are vessels for universal life force."

53. "My mind, body, and spirit feed on positive energy."

54. "I and I alone control how I feel. I always choose to feel positivity and happiness, even when life seems difficult."

55. "I strongly believe in my abilities. The only person I compare myself to is the person I was yesterday."

56. "Creative energies surge through me every moment of the day and bring with them tons of new, creative ideas for my life, business, and career."

57. "Happiness and positivity are choices I choose to experience every minute of my waking life."

58. "I possess an innately developed ability to overcome negative thoughts, conquer my fears, and surpass my limits."

59. "I am a loved child of the universe. The universe always works to ensure my overall wellbeing."

60. "Everything that happens to me has a purpose. In as much as it happens to me, it happens for me too."

When it comes to positive affirmations, remember to keep in mind that they should be just that: positive. This, therefore, means that as you create affirmations for positivity (to enhance your positive thinking and foster an optimistic mindset), you should present-orient your affirmations and make sure the wording is also positive.

Affirmations for Improved Self-Image

Poor self-image (or body image) develops out of a hate for oneself. At its very heart, a poor self-image is a symptom of self-hate. Self-hate is a negative character trait that you can counter with positive affirmation geared towards improving your relationship with your body.

The following affirmations will help improve self-image

61. "I am beautifully and wonderfully created."

62. "I am perfect just as I am right now."

63. "I am an attractive person who attracts positive people and creates favorable circumstances in my life."

64. "I always look and feel great."

65. "My body is on a temple on which I pour love, care, and affection."

66. "I am a confident person admired by many."

67. "I am a strong and capable person. I can overcome anything life throws at me."

68. "Each moment of each day is an opportunity for self-love and care."

69. "I embrace my faults."

70. "I am deserving of love."

71. "I believe in myself and my abilities."

72. "I am very proud of the person I am right now and the person I am becoming."

73. "I deserve happiness and success."

74. "I always do my best."

75. "I am a change catalyst. I adapt well to change."

76. "I see negative criticism for what it is: one person's opinion."

77. "I accept and love myself as I am right now."

78. "My imperfections are what make me unique and one of a kind."

79. "I treat everyone with love and kindness, and everyone reciprocates in kind."

80. "I let go of all negative thoughts about my body, my abilities, and accept positivity as my destiny."

A positive self-image leads to improved confidence. With that said, you can also create affirmations specifically meant to improve your confidence.

Chapter 7: Guided Meditation for Weight Loss

Before you can begin using meditations to do things such as help you burn fat, you need to make sure that you set yourself up correctly for your meditation sessions. Each meditation is going to consist of you entering a deep state of relaxation, following guided hypnosis, and then awakening yourself out of this state of relaxation. If done correctly, you will find yourself experiencing the stages of changed mindset and changed behavior that follows the session.

To properly set yourself up for a meditation experience, you need to make sure that you have a quiet space where you can engage in your meditation. You want to be as uninterrupted as possible so that you do not stir awake from your meditation session. Aside from having a quiet space, you should also make sure that you are comfortable in the area that you will be in. For some of the meditations, I will share, you can be lying down or doing this meditation before bed so that the information sinks in as you sleep. For others, you are going to want to be sitting upright, ideally with your legs crossed on the floor, or with your feet planted on the floor as you sit in a chair. Staying in a sitting position, especially during morning meditations, will help you stay awake and increase your motivation. Laying down during these meditations earlier in the day may result in you draining your energy and feeling completely exhausted, rather than motivated. As a result, you may work against what you are trying to achieve.

Each of these meditations is going to involve a visualization practice; however, if you find that visualization is generally difficult for you, you can listen. The key here is to make sure that you keep as open of a mind as possible so that you can stay receptive to the information coming through these guided meditations.

Aside from all of the above, listening to low music, using a pillow or a small blanket, and dressing in comfortable loose clothing will all help you have better meditations. You want to make sure that you make these experiences the best possible so that you look forward to them and regularly engage in them. As well, the more

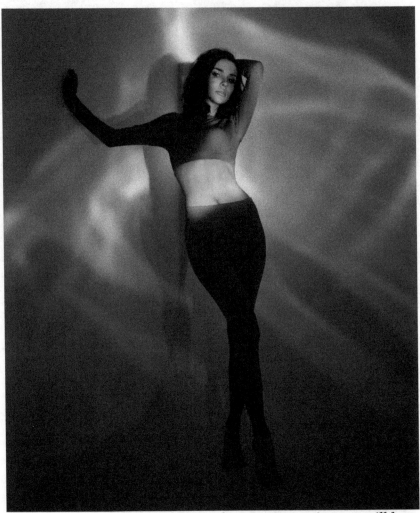

relaxed and comfortable you are, the more receptive you will be to the information being provided to you within each meditation.

A Simple Daily Weight Loss Meditation

This meditation is an excellent simple meditation for you to use daily. It is a short meditation that will not take more than about 15 minutes to complete, and it will provide you with excellent motivation to stick to your weight loss regimen every single day. You should schedule time in your morning routine to engage in this simple daily weight loss meditation every single day. You can also complete it periodically throughout the day if you find your motivation dwindling or your mindset regressing. Over time, you should find that using it just once per day is plenty.

Because you are using this medication in the morning, make sure that you are sitting upright with a straight spine so that you can stay engaged and awake throughout the entire meditation. Laying down or getting too comfortable may result in you feeling more tired, rather than more awake, from your meditation. Ideally, this meditation should lead to boosted energy as well as improved fat burning abilities within your body.

The Meditation

Start by gently closing your eyes and drawing your attention to your breath. As you do, I want you to track the next five breaths, gently and intentionally lengthening them to help you relax as deeply as you can.

Now that you are starting to feel more relaxed, I want you to draw your awareness into your body. First, become aware of your feet. Feel your feet relaxing deeply, as you visualize any stress or worry melting away from your feet. Now, become aware of your legs. Feel any stress or worry melting away from your legs as they begin to relax completely. Next, become aware of your glutes and pelvis, allowing any stress or worry to fade away as they completely relax. Now, relax your entire torso, allowing any stress or anxiety to melt away from your body as it relaxes completely. Next, become aware of your shoulders, arms, hands, and fingers. Allow the stress and worry to melt away from your shoulders, arms, hands, and fingers as they relax entirely. Now, let the stress and fear melt away from your neck, head, and face. Feel your neck, head, and face relaxing as any stress or anxiety melts away completely.

As you deepen into this state of relaxation, I want you to take a moment to visualize the space in front of you. Imagine that in front of you, you are standing there looking back at yourself. See every inch of your body as it is right now standing before you, casually, as you observe yourself. While you do, see what parts of your body you want to reduce fat in so that you can create a healthier, stronger body for yourself. Visualize the fat in these areas of your body, slowly fading away as you begin to carve out a more robust, leaner, and stronger body underneath. Notice how effortlessly this extra fat melts away as you continue to visualize yourself becoming a healthier and more vivacious version of yourself.

Now, I want you to visualize what this healthier, leaner version of yourself would be doing. Visualize yourself going through your typical daily routine, except the perspective of your healthier self. What would you be eating? When and how would you be exercising? What would you spend your time doing? How do you feel about yourself? How different do you feel when you interact with the people around you, such as your family and your co-workers? What does life feel like when you are a healthier, leaner version of you?

Spend several minutes visualizing how different your life is now that your fat has melted away. Feel how natural it is for you to enjoy these healthier foods, and how easy it is for you to moderate your cravings and indulgences when you choose to treat yourself. Notice how easy it is for you to engage in exercise and how exercise feels enjoyable and like a beautiful hobby, rather than a chore that you have to force yourself to commit to every single day. Feel yourself genuinely enjoying life far more, all because the unhealthy fats that were weighing you down and disrupting your health have faded away. Notice how easy it was for you to get here, and how easy it is for you to continue to maintain your health and wellness as you continue to choose better and better choices for you and your body.

Feel how much you respect your body when you make these healthier choices, and how much you genuinely care about yourself. Notice how each meal and each exercise feels like an act of self-care, rather than a chore you are forcing yourself to engage in. Feel how good it feels to do something for you and your wellbeing.

When you are ready, take that visualization of yourself and send the image out far, watching it become nothing more than a spec in your field of awareness. Then, send it out into the ether, trusting that your subconscious mind will hold onto this vision of yourself and work daily on bringing this version of you into your current reality.

Now, awaken back into your body where you sit right now. Feel yourself feeling more motivated, more energized, and more excited about engaging in the activities that are going to improve your health and help you burn your fat. As you prepare to go about your day, hold onto that visualization and those feelings that you had of yourself, and trust that you can have this enjoyable experience in your life. You can do it!

Chapter 8: Daily Weight Loss Meditation

Meditation is in fashion. As soon as you tell someone that you have a problem, it is a rare occasion when they do not recommend you practice it. It does not matter if the problem is mental or physical.

Sometimes, people's insistence leads us to reject a plan idea. However, would it not be more interesting to ask why so many people agree to advise you the same thing?

Interest in Eastern cultures brought the influence of ideas to the forefront. And they are our existence's nucleus. Nutrition and physical exercise promote our body's optimal working.

Yet it is also true that when our emotions aren't controlled, the brain secretes substances that affect our body and mind.

Therefore, physical sufferings or thoughts that make life difficult for us can appear. In this way, meditation helps to keep us safe.

Meditation lowered inflammation levels

Beyond what happened in mind, they find an inflammation measure lower than before the investigation. It indicates that perception benefits go beyond what would appear.

The group manager warns that the exact extent of its benefits cannot yet be defined. Nevertheless, the observation is adequate to multiply scientists' efforts in this regard.

It is no longer about Buddhist experiences or self-help customers who can't control.

We have evidence. However, intentional meditation enhances our quality of life. Furthermore, the fact that its effects last four months means that it is a long-term practice that benefits us.

Given the number of harmful elements to which we are exposed, without being able to do anything, it seems reasonable to bet on this option.

All this shows us how the first step to improving our health is to listen to our bodies.

It is very unlikely that the affects you notice when introducing a new habit constitute a mere imagination. Therefore, from here, we want to thank the efforts of many people who have defended an alternative lifestyle—another class of medicine.

Even when they have been treated as "enlightened" and little sane, their constancy and the defense of their values have been translated into a scientific study that has proved them right and from which we will all benefit.

Practicing anti-stress meditation at home

We know that sometimes it costs. How to combine our daily obligations with that moment of anti-stress meditation? We get up with things to do and arrive at bed with a mind full of those tasks and commitments that must be fulfilled for the following day.

Be careful if the preceding paragraph is an example of what you always live in your day today. It is essential that you know how to organize times and set limits, control all those pressures that do not allow you to get rest.

Ideally, you learn to balance your life. Where you are always the priority of taking care of your health and your emotions, stress can hurt you a lot, and you should see it as an enemy to dominate, to do small to be able to handle it properly. We explain how to practice anti-stress meditation.

1. Emotional agenda

Do you keep an agenda in your day to day of the things you should do? Of your obligations, appointments, meetings, appointments with teachers of children, or your visit to the doctor?

Do the same with your emotions, with your personal needs. Spend at least one hour or two hours for yourself each day. To do what you like, to be alone, and to practice anti-stress meditation. Your emotions have priority, make a hole in your day today. You deserve it, and you need it.

2. A moment of tranquility

It doesn't matter where it is. In your room, in the kitchen or in a park. You must be calm and surrounded by an environment that is pleasant, placid, and comforting. If you want, put on the music that you like, but you must be alone.

3. Regulate your breathing

Let's now take care of our breathing. Once you are comfortable, start to take a deep breath through your nose. Allow your chest to swell, then let this air out little by little through your mouth. If you repeat it six or seven times, you will begin to notice a comforting tingling through your body, and you feel better and calmer.

4. Focus thoughts

What will we do after? Visualize those pressures that concern you most. Are you pressured at work? Do you have problems with your partner? Visualize those images and keep breathing. The tension should soften, the nerves should lose their intensity, and the fear will soften. You will feel better little by little.

5. Positive images

Once you have focused those images, what more pressure they cause on your being, let's now go on to visualize pleasant things, aspects that you would like to be living, and that would make you happy.

They must be simple things: a walk on the beach, you touching the bark of a tree, you walk through a quiet city where the sun illuminates your face and where the rumor of nearby coffee shops envelops you with a pleasant smell of coffee... Easy things, make you happy. Visualize it and keep breathing deeply.

6. The silence

Now we close our eyes. At least for two minutes. Try not to think about anything; just let the silence envelop you. You are at peace, and you are well, there is no pressure. There are only you and a quiet world where there are no pressures and threats, and everything is warm and pleasant.

7. Open your eyes in a renewed way

It is time to open your eyes and breathe normally again. Look around without moving, without getting up. Don't do it, or you'll run the risk of getting dizzy. Allow about five minutes to pass before you walk again. Surely you feel much better, lighter, and without any pressure on your body.

8. New perspectives

Now that you feel more relaxed, try to think about what you can do to find yourself better day by day. Being a little happier sometimes requires that we have to make small changes. And the good thing about anti-stress meditation is that it is slowly changing us inside.

It requires us to make small changes to find the balance so that the body and the mind feel in tune again, and the pressures, the anxieties go out of our body like the smoke that escapes through a window.

Simple Meditation Exercises

Stress accumulates like oil. Paradoxically, as one increases, the other declines. Therefore, stress and energy can fuel a wide variety of sources. For example, stress may feed on problems in various places, or simply a life pattern marked by lack of breaks. We will present simple meditation exercises to help relieve this stress.

Indeed, meditation encourages self-awareness. It is an ancient India peculiar millennial technique, popular in Buddhist and Hindu beliefs. It's become common in the West in recent years.

Some of the advantages of meditation is an increase in the ability to focus, which is the starting point for many other advantages, such as better memory. This also usually enables physical and emotional relaxation. This may also improve our immune system against threats to our safety.

Without further explanation, let's add a set of basic meditation exercises that we can put into action to optimize its benefits.

1. Focus your attention on breathing

The first of the simple meditation exercises is also one of the easiest to incorporate into our routine. We will do it more easily if we can adopt a relaxed position with semi-open eyes.

It is also good to focus on our breathing without trying to vary the parameters. It's about perceiving the air coming in and going out. At this moment, it is common to be distracted by different thoughts. Our mission will be to ignore them until they lose their strength.

2. Countdown

This technique is extremely simple and is of great use when it comes to meditating. With your eyes closed, count back from high numbers such as 50 or 100 until you reach zero. The goal of this practice is to focus our attention on a single thought/activity. In this way, we will be able to eliminate the sensations produced by the rest of the stimulations.

3. Scan our own body

This is the most interesting one of many and simple meditation exercises. We only need to reassess the different parts of our body. For this, it is recommended to place ourselves in a place of weak stimulation. Then we will focus our attention on all parts of our body, starting from the head to finish with the feet.

We can contract and release the different muscle groups to become aware of their presence and their movement. It is a rather attractive way to observe ourselves and to perceive in detail the sensations of our body.

4. Observe dynamically

This exercise is focused on studying our climate. Let's start with a comfortable position; the best is sitting with your eyes closed. We'll then open them to close them for a moment. Before that, we'll have to focus on what's learned.

We'll be able to think about the various sensations that we're generating the stimulations that came to us. We may list them; think of each object's shapes and colors, or name. Furthermore, if we know this at home, it might be a good way to experience our home differently.

5. Meditating in motion

Another basic meditation exercise we can put into action is based on our body's feedback of fun stimuli as it moves. For this, interaction with nature is recommended.

For example, we can take a few steps on the beach or in the woods and enjoy the warmth of the sun on our face, the wind caresses, or the touch of plants and water on our hands. It can also be another way to make a personal observation, thinking about our body's movements as we walk.

6. Meditate with fire

Finally, we can use fire as a symbolic purification item to focus our meditation. We may concentrate on a campfire in nature or something simpler: a candle's flame. It will allow us to experience the heat sensations associated with fire and the shadows reflecting on the surrounding objects.

On the other side, we can list and burn negative items in our everyday lives. This positive gesture that can be performed symbolically or factually helps us free ourselves from our worries of something we have no influence over.

Chapter 9: Hypnosis to Stop Emotional Eating

What Is Emotional Eating?

People usually eat to beat physical hunger. However, some people are relying on food as a source of comfort or addressing their negative emotions. Some also use food as a reward whenever they achieve their goals or when celebrating special events like birthdays or weddings.

When you use food as a cover or a solution for extreme emotions, then you suffer from emotional eating. The feelings that trigger your eating are mostly negative, for example, stress, loneliness, sadness, or when you are grieving. However, it is not only the negative emotions that can cause emotional eating; some positive emotions such as happiness or feelings of comfort can also trigger emotional eating.

There is a difference in the way people use food to address their emotions. While some people rely on food when they are in the middle of their life situations, others may find comfort in food soon after the situation is over. They use food as a recovery tool.

A problem associated with emotional eating is that it may prevent you from utilizing other adaptive approaches to problems. You should also know that emotional eating does not solve the issues you are going through. If anything, it only serves to make you feel worse. After eating, the original emotional problem remains unsolved, and on top of it, you find yourself feeling guilty of overeating. It is, therefore, essential for you to identify the problem of emotional eating and to take timely appropriate measures to stop it.

How to Recognize Emotional Eating

The best way for you to know if you are suffering from emotional eating is to find out whether you always eat because you are hungry, or you eat impulsively. You should pay attention to your emotions and how you usually cope with them. Find out if you are utilizing food just for hunger or you are unconsciously overeating.

Once you are sure you have an emotional eating problem, take appropriate steps to stop it. This is because not all the food you eat is healthy. You will occasionally find yourself eating unhealthy food such as junk food and sweets, which could be detrimental to your health.

Common Features of Emotional Hunger

It is easy for you to mistake emotional hunger for normal physical hunger. You, therefore, need to learn how to make a distinction between the two forms of hunger. The following are some of the hints you can use to tell the difference between the two kinds of hunger:

Emotional Hunger Comes Unexpectedly

You tend to experience emotional hunger suddenly. The feelings of craving will then overwhelm you, forcing you to look for food urgently. On the other hand, feelings of physical hunger tend to grow gradually. Also, when you are physically hungry, you will not be overwhelmed suddenly by hunger, not unless you have gone for days without food.

Emotional Hunger Desires for Some Specific Food

If you are physically hungry, any food is right for you. Physical hunger is not too selective on the type of food to consume. You will feel satisfied eating healthy food like fruits and vegetables. On the other hand, emotional hunger tends to be selective on the food to consume. In most cases, emotional hunger craves unhealthy foods, such as sweets, snacks, and junk food. The craving for these foods tends to be overwhelming and urgent. You may experience strong desires for such food as pizza or cheesecake, and you have no appetite for any other type of food.

Emotional Eating Lacks Concern for Consequences

If you are involved in emotional eating, then in most cases, you find yourself eating without any concern about the consequences of overeating on your general wellbeing. You also eat without paying attention to the food you are consuming. You are not concerned about the quality of the food or its nutritional value. All you care about is the quantity of the food to satisfy your craving. Your goal will be to eat as much food as possible.

On the other hand, when you are eating because of physical hunger, you will be conscious of the quality and the quantity of food you are consuming. You will be concern about the health benefits of the food you are eating. You will also choose to eat a very well-balanced diet, which will prevent your body from overeating junk foods.

Emotional Hunger Is Insatiable

If you are suffering from emotional eating, your hunger cannot be satisfied no matter the amount of food you have consumed. Hunger as a craving will refuse to get out of your mind. You will keep craving for more and more food, and soon, you will find yourself eating continuously without a break.

On the other hand, physical hunger is satisfied the moment your stomach is full. You may experience feelings of physical hunger only during specific times of the day. This could be the response of your body once you have conditioned it to receive food at times of the day.

Emotional Hunger Is Located on Your Mind

Unlike physical hunger, the craving for food originates from your mind. Emotional hunger involves the obsession originating from your mind on some specific type of food. You find yourself unable to ignore or overcome this obsession. You then give in to it and reach for your favorite food.

On the other hand, physical hunger originates from the stomach. You feel the hunger pang from your stomach. You can also occasionally feel growling from your belly whenever you are hungry.

Emotional Hunger Comes with Guilt and Regrets

When you are suffering from emotional eating, deep down, you know your eating does not come with any nutritional benefits. You will then have feelings of guilt or even shame. You know you are doing your health a lot of harm and you may start regretting your actions. On the other hand, physical eating involves eating to satisfy your hunger. You will not suffer any feelings of shame or guilt for meeting your bodily needs.

Causes of Your Emotional Eating

For you to succeed in putting a stop to your emotional eating habits, you need to find out what triggers them. Find out the exact situations, feelings, or places that make you feel like eating whenever you are exposed to. Below are some of the common causes of emotional eating:

Stress

One symptom of stress is hunger. You tend to experience the feeling of hunger whenever you are stressed. When you are stressed, your body responds by producing a stress hormone known as Cortisol. When this hormone is produced in high quantities, it will trigger a craving for foods that are salty or sugary in nature as well as any fried food. These are the food which gives you a lot of instant energy and pleasure.

If you do not control stress in your life, you will always be seeking relief in unhealthy food.

Boredom

You could be eating to relieve yourself of boredom. You can also resort to eating to beat idleness. Besides, you may be using food to occupy your time because you do not have much to do. Food can also fill your void and momentarily distract you from the hidden feelings of directionless and dissatisfaction with yourself. Whenever you feel purposeless, you tend to reach out for food to make you feel better. However, the truth is that food can never be a solution to any of your negative emotions.

Childhood Habits

Emotional eating could be a result of your childhood habits. For example, if your parents used to reward your good behaviors with foods such as sweets, ice cream, or pizza, you may have carried these habits to your adulthood. You will find yourself rewarding yourself with your childhood snack whenever you accomplish a given task. You can also be unconsciously eating because of the nostalgic feelings of your childhood. This happens when you always cherish the delicacies you used to eat in your childhood. Food can also serve as a powerful reminder of your most cherished childhood memories, for example, if you were eating cookies with your dad during your outings together. Whenever you miss your dad, your first instinct is to reach out for the cookies.

Social Influences

Occasionally, you may need to go out with your friends and have a good time. During such outings, you can share a meal to relieve stress. However, such social events can lead to overeating. You can find yourself overeating at the nudge of your close friends or family who encourages you to go for an extra serving. It is easy to fall into their temptation.

Avoiding Emotions

You may use eating as a way of temporarily avoiding the emotions you are feeling, such as the feeling of anxiety, shame, resentment, or anger. Eating is a perfect way to prevent negative distractions, albeit temporarily.

Habits and Practices, You Can Use to Overcome Emotional Eating to Lose Weight

Practice Healthy Lifestyle Habits

You will handle life's shortcomings better when you are physically strong, happy, and well-rested. However, if you are exhausted, any stressful situation you encounter will trigger the craving for food. In this regard, you need to make physical exercise part of your daily routine. You also need to have enough time to sleep to feel rested. Moreover, engage yourself in social activities with others. Create time for outings with family or close friends.

Practice Mindfulness by Eating Slowly

When you eat to satisfy your feelings rather than your stomach, you tend to eat so fast and mindlessly that you fail to savor the taste or texture of your food. However, when you slow down and take a moment to savor every bite, you will be less likely to indulge in overeating. Slowing down also helps you to enjoy your food better.

Accept All Your Feelings

Emotional eating is often triggered by feelings of helplessness over your emotions. You lack the courage to handle your feelings head-on, so you seek refuge in food. However, you need to be mindful of your feelings. Learn to overcome your emotions by accepting them. Once you do this, you regain the courage to handle any feelings that triggers your emotional eating.

Take a Moment Before Giving in to Your Cravings

Typically, emotional eating is sudden and mindless. It takes you by surprise, and often you may feel powerless in stopping the urge to eat. However, you can control the sudden urges to reach for food if you take a moment of 5 minutes before you give in. This allows you a moment to reconsider your decisions and eventually get the craving out of your mind.

Find Other Alternative Solutions to Your Emotion

Actively look for other solutions to address your feelings other than eating. For example, whenever you feel lonely, instead of eating, reach out for your phone and call that person who always puts a smile on your face. Look for good alternatives to food that you can rely on to feel emotionally fulfilled. If you feel anxious, learn to do exercises.

Chapter 10: Eat Healthy with Subliminal Hypnosis

You can also use specific strategies and mental exercises that can help you cut calories and burn fat faster. These six strategies and mindset exercises can help you reinforce the changes you are creating through your daily hypnosis sessions. This way, you are more likely to stay on track longer and increase the amount of time you experience between regression periods.

Affirmations

Affirmations can be an incredible way to keep your mindset focused on a healthy lifestyle. When you are working on changing your subconscious mind, repeating affirmations to yourself can help reinforce the changes you are making during meditations. Affirmations, then, allow you to empower yourself to believe in these changes and continue to adhere to them as you go along in life. Some people will use just one or two affirmations, whereas others will have multiple affirmations that they use depending on what situation they are presently in.

Eating with the Right Mindset

When you set aside time to eat during the day, make sure that you are eating with the right mindset. You want to be eating from a place of being genuinely hungry, and you want to eat with the mindset of wanting to nourish your body. If you find yourself eating from the mindset of desperation, cravings, or overwhelming emotions, you will likely find yourself eating foods that are less than healthy for you. You should always take a few moments to ask yourself: "why am I eating?" and "what am I choosing to nourish my body with?" Your answers should be because I am genuinely hungry and with something nutritious.

Short Meditations

Meditations are a great way to help keep you on track with your healthy eating. In this part, we tackled three great shorter meditations that you can use to help you eat healthier foods on a day to day basis. Short meditations are great because they allow you the opportunity to quickly get your mindset back on track and

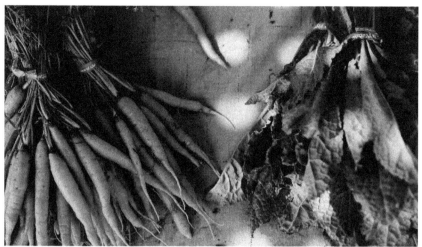

keep yourself focused. They can easily be used in a short period of time to keep yourself focused and eating healthier while supporting your weight loss goals.

Eating Foods, You Enjoy

If you are trying to lose weight through a diet that you genuinely do not enjoy, you are going to have a hard time sticking on your diet. Food is something that has the capacity to give us joy and stimulates our reward center in our brain. This means that every time you eat something you enjoy; you genuinely derive pleasure from it and feel your best. Eating a diet that you do not enjoy essentially robs you of that pleasure, meaning you will be more likely to choose food options that are not great for you. As you work on weight loss, make sure that you are eating healthier foods that you genuinely enjoy so that you are more likely to reach for them over anything else.

Making Eating an Experience

As you eat, make sure that you make eating as an experience. Slow down, indulge in each bite, and strive to taste every single bite you can have. Chew thoroughly and allow yourself to feel completely satisfied with everything you eat. Making eating about the experience rather than about the chore of feeding yourself means that you are more likely to gain pleasure and joy out of what you are eating in the first place. As well, you are more likely to focus on eating only when you are hungry, rather than eating to fill the time or eating because you are feeling emotional.

Mindful Eating

Lastly, engage in mindful eating. When you are using hypnosis and meditation to support you in weight loss, mindful eating is a great practice that goes hand in hand with that. You can help yourself lose weight by intuitively picking your meals and practicing portion control. Rather than letting yourself indulge in habits or in the cravings of your body, let yourself mindfully decide what the best meal option for you is, and what portion you should be eating. Notice when you are full and stop eating and notice when you are hungry and opt for something nutritious. If you notice you have a craving for a certain treat, indulge in a small portion of it to satisfy your craving, rather than strictly denying yourself from it. Following these mindful patterns mean that you will be more likely to stay on track with your weight loss goals, rather than trying to force yourself to stick to habits or eating behaviors that do not feel right for you.

Meditation for Cutting Calories

This meditation is an excellent meditation to help you cut calories, allowing you to decrease the amount of food that you are eating daily. This is a 10-15-minute meditation that will support you in reducing cravings while also reducing your food intake daily. The goal of this particular meditation is to reduce calorie intake without causing you to starve yourself, so the goal will ultimately be to help you choose healthier meals that help you feel fuller longer, while also cutting out unnecessary snacking in between meals.

You should engage in this meditation at the beginning of the day, or any time you feel yourself having trouble with food cravings or moderation. That way, you can encourage yourself to stay on track with your weight loss goals. With that being said, you should make sure that you are sitting up with a straight spine during this particular meditation so that you stay engaged and do not lose your energy or motivation following this particular meditation.

The Meditation

Start this meditation by sitting upright in a comfortable position with your spine long and tall and your awareness soft and gentle. When you are ready, I want you to begin to draw your awareness into the center of your chest, directly behind your sternum. As you do, notice how it rises and falls with each breath you take. As you breathe in, feel your sternum pushing away from your spine, and as you breathe out, feel it falling back toward your spine. Continue to focus on this space for four breaths as you relax into this position and enjoy your meditation.

When you start to feel yourself relaxing, I want you to start visualizing yourself, putting together a meal for yourself. Start with breakfast. See yourself filling your plate with healthy options that fill you up without wasting calories. Notice how easy it is to fill your plate with things that are healthy for you, and that helps you feel your best. Allow yourself to begin feeling excited about the food options on that plate, noticing that you are genuinely craving them and looking forward to this meal. Visualize yourself taking a bite of the food and imagine how amazing it tastes. Notice how you feel yourself being completely satisfied with this food and that you do not have any reason to snack on anything in between because you are so content with your meal.

When it does come time to have a snack, or your following meal, see yourself having the desire to indulge in something healthy again. Notice how easy it is for you to pass up on junk foods or foods that do not support your health because you genuinely enjoy eating things that are healthier for you. See yourself easily opting for healthier food choices and enjoying each food option that you choose. Feel how great it is that being healthy, cutting calories, and losing weight can be so delicious.

Now, when you are ready, bring your awareness back into your present body. Feel yourself awakening into your body, coming back into your conscious state of awareness. Then, when you are ready, you can go about your day once again. Feel yourself effortlessly gravitating toward healthier meal options all day as you focus more on what is going to help you feel healthy, satisfied, and fulfilled from your meals.

Chapter 11: Portion Control Hypnosis

Whether you wish to shed many pounds or maintain a healthy weight, proper portion consumption is as necessary as the consumption of appropriate foods. The rate of obesity among youngsters and adults has increased partly owing to the increase in restaurant portions.

A portion is the total quantity of food that you eat in one sitting. A serving size is the suggested quantity of one food. For instance, the amount of steak you eat for dinner maybe a portion; however, three ounces of steak, maybe a serving. Controlling serving sizes helps with portion control.

Health Benefits of Portion Control

Serious health problems are caused by overeating, for example, type 2 diabetes, weight problems, high blood pressure, and many more. Therefore, when you are looking to lead a healthy lifestyle, portion control should be a significant priority.

Fullness and Weight Management

Feeling satiable, or having a sense of fullness, will affect the quantity you eat and the way you usually eat. According to the British Nutrition Foundation, eating smaller portions slowly increases the feeling of satiety after a meal.

Eating smaller parts also permits your body to use the food you eat right away for energy, rather than storing the excess as fat. Losing weight is not as straightforward as solely controlling your portion sizes; however, once you learn to observe the quantity of food you eat, you will begin to apply conscious intake, which might assist you in making healthier food decisions.

When you eat too quickly, you do not notice your stomach's cues that it is full. Eat slowly and listen to hunger cues to enhance feelings of fullness and, ultimately, consume less food.

Improved Digestion

Considerably larger portion sizes contribute to an upset stomach and discomfort (caused by a distended stomach pushing down on

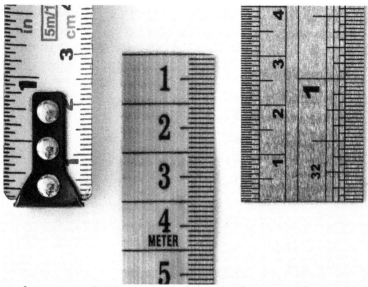

your other organs). Your gastrointestinal system functions best when it is not full of food. Managing portions can help to get rid of cramping and bloating after eating. You furthermore may run the danger of getting pyrosis, because of having a full abdomen will push hydrochloric acid back into your digestive tract.

Money Savings

Eating smaller parts may lead to monetary benefits, mainly when eating out. In addition to eating controlled serving sizes, you do not have to purchase as many groceries. Measuring serving proportions can make the box of cereal and packet of nuts last longer than eating straight out of the container.

Take, for instance, the method to apply portion management at restaurants is to order kid-sized meals, that are typically cheaper than adult meals and closer to the right serving size you ought to be eating.

Adult portion sizes at restaurants will equal two, three, or even more servings. Therefore, immediately the food arrives at your table, request for a takeaway container and put away half of your food from the plate. Take your food home and this way, you will have two meals for the worth of one.

How to Control Portions Using Hypnosis

Hypnosis can take you into a deeply relaxed state and quickly train your mind to understand when to do away with excess food instinctively, and allow your digestion to be lighter, and more comfortable. You may discover the pleasure of being in tune with what your own body requires nourishment. Hypnosis will re-educate your instincts to regulate hunger pangs. As you relax and repeatedly listen to powerful hypnotic suggestions that are going to be absorbed by your mind; you may quickly begin to note that:

- Your mind is no longer engrossed in food
- Your abdomen and gut feel lighter
- You now do not feel uncontrollable hunger pangs at 'non-meal' times
- You naturally forget to have food between meals
- You begin to enjoy a healthier lifestyle

There is a somewhat simple self-hypnosis process for helping you control your appetite and portions. In a shell, you are immersing yourself into psychological state and picture a dial, or a flip switch of some type that is symbolic of your craving and your real hunger. Then you repeatedly apply to develop a true sense of control, then you employ it out of the hypnotic state and when confronted with those things and circumstances to curb the perceived hunger and control your appetite.

Step 1: Get yourself into a comfortable position and one where you will remain undisturbed for the period of this exercise. Ascertain your feet are flat on the ground and hands not touching. Then once you are in position, calm yourself.

You can do that by using hypnosis tapes; they are basic processes to assist you in opening the door of your mind.

Step 2: You may prefer to deepen your hypnotic state. The best and most straightforward is imagining yourself in your favorite place and relaxing your body bit by bit. Keep focused on the session at hand (that is, watch out to not drift off) then go to the third step.

Step 3: Take a picture of a dial, a lever or a flippy switch of some kind that is on a box or mounted on a wall of some sort, let it fully controls your mind's eye. Notice the colors, the materials that it is created out of, and the way it indicates 0-10 to mark the variable degrees of your real hunger.

Notice wherever it is indicating currently let it show you how hungry you are. Remember when last you ate, what you ate, whether the hunger is genuine or merely reacting to a recent bout of gluttony and wanting to gratify that sensation!

Once you have established the dial, where it is set, and trusting that the reading is correct, then go to the subsequent step.

Step 4: Flip the dial down a peg and notice the effects taking place within you. Study your feedback and ascertain that it feels like you are moving your appetite with the dial. The more you believe you are affecting your appetite with the dial, the more practical its application in those real-life situations.

Practice turning it down even lower and start recognizing how you use your mind to change your perceived appetite utilizing a method that is healthy and helps keep you alert when you encounter circumstances with plenty of food supply. Tell yourself that the more you observe this, the better control you gain over your appetite.

You might even create a strong affirmation that accompanies this dial "I am in control of my eating" is one such straightforward statement. Word it as you wish and make sure it is one thing that resonates well with you. Once you have repeated the meaningful affirmations to yourself severally with conviction, proceed to the following step.

Step 5: Visualize yourself during a future scenario, where there is going to be constant temptation to continue eating although you are full, or to consume an excessive amount. See the sights of that place, take a mental note of the other people there, notice the smells, hear the sounds. Become increasingly aware of how you are feeling in this place. Get the most definition and clarity possible, then notice that once the temptation presents itself, you turn down the dial on your craving. You realize that you are not hungry to eat anymore, then repeat your positive affirmations to yourself a few more times to strengthen it.

Run through this future situation severally on loop to make sure your mind is mentally rehearsed about your plan to respond.

Step 6: Twitch your little finger and toes, then open your eyes and proceed to observe your skills in real-life and spot how much control you have.

Chapter 12: The Power of Repeated Words and Thoughts

Hypnosis is rewiring your brain to add or to change your daily routine starting from your basic instincts. This happens due to the fact that while you are in a hypnotic state, you are more susceptible to suggestions by the person who put you in this state. In the case of self-hypnosis, the person who made you enter the trance of hypnotism is yourself. Thus, the only person who can give you suggestions that can change your attitude in this method is you and you alone.

Again, you must forget the misconception that hypnosis is like sleeping because if it is then it would be impossible to give autosuggestions to yourself. Try to think about it like being in a very vivid daydream where you are capable of controlling every aspect of the situation you are in. This gives you the ability to change anything that may bother and hinder you to achieve the best possible result. If you are able to pull it off properly, then the possibility of improving yourself after the constant practice of the method will just be a few steps away.

Career

People say that motivation is the key to improve in your career. But no matter how you love your career, you must admit that there are aspects of your work that you really do not like doing. Even if it is a fact that you are good in the other tasks, there is that one duty that you dread. And every time you encounter this specific chore you seem to be slowed down and thus lessening your productivity at work. This is where self-hypnosis comes into play.

The first thing you need to do is find that task you do not like. In some cases, there might be multiple of them depending on your personality and how you feel about your job. Now, try to look at why you do not like that task and do simple research on how to make the job a lot simpler. You can then start conditioning yourself to use the simple method every time you do the job.

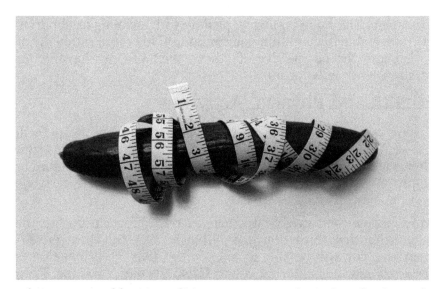

After you are able to condition your state of mind to do the task, each time you encounter it will become the trigger for your trance and thus giving you the ability to perform it better. You will not be able to tell the difference since you will not mind it at all. Your coworkers and superiors though will definitely notice the change in your work style and in your productivity.

Family

It is easy to improve in a career. But to improve your relationship with your family can be a little trickier. Yet, self-hypnosis can still reprogram you to interact with your family members better by modifying how you react to the way they act. You will have the ability to adjust your way of thinking, depending on the situation. This then allows you to respond in the most positive way possible no matter how dreadful the scenario may be.

If you are in a fight with your husband/wife, for example, the normal reaction is to flare up and face fire with fire. The problem with this approach is it usually engulfs the entire relationship, which might eventually lead up to separation. Being in a hypnotic state in this instance then can help you think clearly and change the impulse of saying words without thinking them through. Anger will still be there, of course, that is the healthy way. But anger now under self-hypnosis can be channeled and stop being a raging inferno, you can turn it into a steady bonfire that can help you and your partner find common ground for whatever issue you are facing. The same applies to dealing with a sibling or children. If you are able to condition your mind to think more rationally or to get into the perspective of others, then you can have better family/friends' relationships.

Health and Physical Activities

Losing weight can be the most common reason why people will use self-hypnosis in terms of health and physical activities. But this is just one part of it. Self-hypnosis can give you a lot more to improve this aspect of your life. It works the same way while working out.

Most people tend to give up their exercise program due to the exhaustion they think they can no longer take. But through self-hypnosis, you will be able to tell yourself that the exhaustion is lessened and thus allowing you to finish the entire routine. Keep in mind though that your mind must never be conditioned to forget exhaustion, it must only not mind it until the end of the exercise. Forgetting it completely might lead you to not stopping to work out until your energy is depleted. It becomes counterproductive in this case.

Having a healthy diet can also be influenced by self-hypnosis. Conditioning your mind to avoid unhealthy food can be done. Thus, hypnosis will be triggered each you are tempted to eat a meal you are conditioned to consider as unhealthy. Your eating habit then can change to benefit you to improve your overall health.

Mental, Emotional and Spiritual Needs

Since self-hypnosis deals directly in how you think, it is then no secret that it can greatly improve your mental, emotional and spiritual needs. A clear mind can give your brain the ability to have more rational thoughts. Rationality then leads to better decision making and easy absorption and retention of the information you might need to improve your mental capacity. You must set your expectations, though; this does not work like magic that can turn you into a genius. The process takes time depending on how far you want to go, how much you want to achieve. Thus, the effects will only be limited by how much you are able to condition your mind.

In terms of emotional needs, self-hypnosis cannot make you feel differently in certain situations. But it can condition you to take in each scenario a little lighter and make you deal with them better. Others think that getting rid of emotion can be the best course of action if you are truly able to rewire your brain. But they seem to forget that even though rational thinking is often influenced negatively by emotion, it is still necessary for you to decide on things basing on the common ethics and aesthetics of the real world. Self-hypnosis then can channel your emotion to work in a more positive way in terms of decision making and dealing with emotional hurdles and problems.

Spiritual need, on the other hand, is far easier to influence when it comes to doing self-hypnosis. As a matter of fact, most people with spiritual beliefs are able to do self-hypnosis each time they practice what they believe in. A deep prayer, for instance, is a way to self-hypnotize yourself to enter the trance to feel closer to a Divine existence. Chanting and meditation done by other religions also leads and have the same goal. Even the songs during a mass or praise and worship triggers self-hypnosis, depending if the person allows them to do so.

Still, the improvements can only be achieved if you condition yourself that you are ready to accept them. The willingness to put an effort must also be there. An effortless hypnosis will only create the illusion that you are improving and thus will not give you the satisfaction of achieving your goal in reality.

How hypnosis can help resolve childhood issues

Another issue that hypnosis can help are problems from our past. If you have had traumatic situations from your childhood days, then you may have issues in all areas of your adult life. Unresolved issues from your past can lead to anxiety and depression in your later years. Childhood trauma is dangerous because it can alter many things in the brain, both psychologically and chemically.

The most vital thing to remember about trauma from your childhood is that given a harmless and caring environment in which the child's vital needs for physical safety, importance, emotional security and attention are met, the damage that trauma and abuse cause can be eased and relieved. Safe and dependable relationships are also a dynamic component in healing the effects of childhood trauma in adulthood and make an atmosphere in which the brain can safely start the process of recovery.

Pure Hypnoanalysis is the lone most effective method of treatment available in the world today for the resolution of phobias, anxiety, depression, fears, psychological and emotional problems/symptoms and eating disorders. It is a highly advanced form of hypnoanalysis (referred to as analytical hypnotherapy or hypno-analysis). Hypnoanalysis, in its numerous forms, is practiced all over the world; this method of hypnotherapy can completely resolve the foundation of anxieties in the unconscious mind, leaving the individual free of their symptoms for life.

There is a deeper realism active at all times around us and inside us. This reality commands that we must come to this world to find happiness, and every so often that our inner child stands in our way. This is by no means intentional; however, it desires to reconcile wounds from the past or address damaging philosophies that were troubling to us as children.

So to disengage the issues that upset us from earlier in our lives we have to find a way to bond with our internal child, we then need to assist in rebuilding this part of us which will, in turn, help us to be rid of all that has been hindering us from moving on.

Connecting with your inner child may seem like something that may be hard or impossible to do, especially since they may be a part that has long been buried. It is a fairly easy exercise to do and can even be done right now. You will need about 20 minutes to complete this exercise. Here's what you do: find a quiet spot where you won't be disturbed and find a picture of you as a child if you think it may help.

Breathe in and loosen your clothing if you have to. Inhale deeply into your abdomen and exhale, repeat until you feel yourself getting relaxed; you may close your eyes and focus on getting less tense. Feel your forehead and head relax, let your face become relaxed and relax your shoulders. Allow your body to be limp and loose while you breathe slowly. Keep breathing slowly as you let all of your tension float away.

Now slowly count from 10 to 0 in your mind and try to think of a place from your childhood. The image doesn't have to be crystal clear right now, but try to focus on exactly how you remember it and keep that image in mind. Imagine yourself as a child and imagine observing younger you; think about your clothes, expression, hair, etc. In your mind go and meet yourself, introduce yourself to you.

Chapter 13: Positive Affirmations

In personal development, an affirmation is a form of autosuggestion in which a statement of a desirable intention is repeated to implant it in the mind. An affirmation is the same, but it is asked as a question because the subconscious loves questions and finds ways to answer them.

Louise Hay, who wrote "You can heal your life," advocates affirmations for every area in life from health to work to home. Louise Hay believes that we cause our illnesses and with the use of affirmations, we can begin the self-healing process.

Louise Hay's explanation for Bell's palsy is 'total unspoken rage.' When I was aged 20, my parents were moving to a new house and insisted that I went with them. I tried extremely hard to refuse but was soon cowed by my mother, who insisted that I would be 'out on the streets' if I didn't move with them. On the morning of the move, I woke up with severe Bell's palsy. I ended up having an operation which involved shaving off most of my hair and cutting off my ear for the surgeon to scrape the nerve causing the palsy. This, in fact, put me more into the clutches of my mother as I had an incredibly crooked face for two years and no hair! When I read 'total unspoken rage,' I knew that was exactly how I felt. From that moment, on I realized that we did cause our own illnesses, we just had to realize it.

I think everyone needs a copy of Louise Hay's books for reference as she talks about how to phrase the affirmations and how often to repeat them. You must always repeat an affirmation at least three times at once and this set must then be repeated several times during the day. Remember, it is repetition that you need but do not include more than three positives in one statement. When I was doing a replacement, I wanted to put:

'I am beautiful, slim, fit, healthy, wealthy and successful'

But with my teacher, we changed it to:

'I am slim, healthy and fit'

The subconscious also strips out the word NOT, so it should never be in an affirmation statement. Using the example above, 'I am not hungry' becomes 'I am hungry'—another reason for weight gain.

If you give yourself a negative message, do the following:

- Stop and ping your elastic band
- Say CANCEL that last statement immediately
- Immediately repeat a positive affirmation three times

To work, affirmations should be in your own words and must feel real to you. You need to say them out loud in a strong voice and really feel them and mean them. Here are a few examples of affirmations that you could use if you wish to use an affirmation, just say it as a question, for example, 'Why am I so healthy?'

If you feel you are going to cheat:

- 'I'm losing weight now'
- 'I love the feeling of making progress'
- To keep you on the straight and narrow:
- 'I'm getting fitter every day'
- 'I am feeling thinner today'
- 'I am getting slimmer and slimmer every day'
- 'I'm losing weight now'
- 'I look and feel lighter today'
- 'I'm enjoying how I'm feeling now'
- 'I love the feeling of making progress'
- 'I love the food that makes me thin'
- 'I am going to fit into the following size smaller any minute'
- 'I enjoy being healthy'
- 'My body is getting stronger, slimmer, and healthier every day'
- 'I feel so thin inside; my outer is just about to catch up'
- 'My metabolism is burning up all the food I eat'
- 'My weight will stay stable for the rest of my life'
- 'I am powerful'

Saying Affirmations Quickly

Recently a therapist told me of a brilliant way to get the most out of repeating your affirmations. If you are like me, you will have rakes of them, ranging from money to weight to career to health and every time you repeat them it becomes such a mouthful. So, type your affirmations up and give them a number. I then say, "Affirmation 1 will be XXXX" and then repeat this affirmation three times. This affirmation then becomes 'Affirmation 1,' or '1' in my subconscious.

In the future, instead of having to repeat all the affirmation say, 'Affirmation 1,' 'Affirmation 2' etc. They really roll off your tongue and you can ensure that you get multiple repetitions done very quickly and efficiently!

Absorbing the Affirmations Quickly

As you are repeating your affirmation, tap around your scalp just outside and around your right ear (this is called temporal tapping). This helps absorb the affirmations into your brain more quickly than just saying them. You may now apply what you have Learned!

Canceling Negative Statements

Remember, if you say something negative, immediately say "cancel that last statement"—you can say it out loud (if you have made the comment) or under your breath, if someone else has made a negative statement. If it helps, wear an elastic band around your wrist and ping it every time you make a negative statement, it stings and really stops you! It is especially important to remember this technique as very often we say things all the time, which are a habit, such 'I am sorry.' If you want to apologize, say "I apologize" as this has a very different energy to, I am sorry.

These are positive statements to say after canceling a negative statement:

- 'I am healthy and well-nourished'
- 'I love myself; I love my body and my excess fat disappears'
- 'I am my ideal weight'
- 'I enjoy exercising several times a week'

- 'I can say 'no'
- 'My body is nourished'
- 'I am proud of my body'
- 'My metabolism works at 100%'
- 'I am spiritually, emotionally and physically balanced'

Talking About Yourself

So, you might want to talk about yourself with positive beliefs, even if you don't believe them at the time, fake it until you make and in the case of weight problems, think like a slim person. A friend of mine who had put on a lot of weight said that she was surprised when she saw a picture of herself at that time, as she believed she was still slim, so it does work both ways!

Most people who are overweight are normally overly critical and always speak negatively about themselves. They normally suffer from low self-worth and low self-esteem. The result is that, by doing this, they are perpetuating the problem. When you are speaking negatively to yourself, ask yourself if you would speak to a friend like that. The answer most probably will be that you would not, so why on earth are you speaking like that to yourself? Stop it now!

It is almost impossible for your body to change when you keep sending it negative messages. If you say, "I am FAT," you give your body more instruction and energy to BE FAT.

You need to change your chatter from negative to positive even if you do not believe what you are saying. I hear you cry, "How can I be positive when I am fat?" but it is especially important in the re-programming of your subconscious and your cells. Positive affirmations are an excellent way of re-programming and these can be combined with EFTTM for stronger and quicker results.

Change 'I am fat' to 'I am getting slimmer every day'

Change 'I never lose weight' to 'It gets easier every day to lose weight'

Chapter 14: The Habit Changing Method

Take Things Slowly

Eating should not be treated as a race. Eat slowly. This just means that you should take your time in relishing and enjoying your food, it is a healthy thing! So, how long do you have to grind up the food in your mouth? Well, there is no specific time food should be chewed, but 18-25 bites are enough to enjoy the food mindfully. This can be hard at first, mainly if you have been used to speed eating for an exceptionally long time. Why not try some new techniques like using chopsticks when you are accustomed to spoon and fork? Or use your non-dominant hand when eating. These strategies can slow you down and improve your awareness.

Avoid Distractions

To make things simpler for you, just make it a habit of sitting down and staying away from distractions. The handful of nuts that you eat as you walk through the kitchen and the bunch of morning snacks you nibbled while standing in front of your fridge can be hard to recall. According to researchers, people tend to eat more when they are doing other things too. You should, therefore, sit down and focus on your food to prevent mindless eating behaviors.

Savor Every Bite

Do not forget that eating mindfully is not only about enjoying the food you eat, but your health too, and without feeling guilty and uncomfortable. Relishing the sight, taste, and smell of your diet is utterly worth it. This can be so easy if you take things gradually and do not rush to perfection. Make small changes towards awareness until you are a fully mindful eater. So, eat slowly and savor the good food you are eating and the proper nutrition you are giving to your body.

Mind the Presentation

Regardless of how busy you are; it is a good idea to set the table, making sure it looks divine. A lovely set of utensils, placement, and napkin made of eco-friendly cloth material is a perfect reminder that you need to sit down and pay attention when you have your meals.

Plate Your Food

Serving yourself and portioning your food before you bring the plate to the table can help you to consume a modest amount, rather than putting a platter on the table from which to continually replenish. You can do this even with crackers, chips, nuts, and other snack foods. Keep yourself away from the temptation of eating straight from a bag of chips and different types of food. It is also helpful if you resize the bag or place the food in smaller containers so that you can stay aware of the amount of food you are eating. Having a bright idea of how much you have eaten will make you stop eating when you are full, or even sooner.

Always Choose Quality over Quantity

By trying to select smaller amounts of the most beautiful food within your means, you will end up enjoying and feeling satisfied without the chance of overeating. With this, it will be helpful if you spend time preparing your meals using quality and fresh ingredients. Cooking can be a pleasurable and relaxing experience if you only let yourself into it. On top of this, you can achieve the peace of mind that comes from knowing what is in the food you are eating.

Do not Invite Your Thoughts and Emotions to Dinner

Just as there are many other factors that affect our sense of mindful eating, as well as the digestive system; it would come as no surprise that our thoughts and emotions play just as much of an important role.

It happens on the odd occasion that one comes home after a long and tiresome day and you feel somewhat "worked up," irritated and angry. This is when negative and even destructive thoughts creep in while you are having supper.

The best practice would be to avoid this altogether. Therefore, if you are feeling unhappy or angry in any way, go for a walk before supper, play with your children, or play with your family pet. But, whatever you do, take your mind off your negative emotions before you attempt to have a meal.

Make a Good Meal Plan for Each Week

When you start the diet, it is advised to stick to the meal plan that comes with the diet. There should be a meal plan of 2 weeks or 4 weeks attached to the diet's guideline. Once you are familiar with the food list, prohibited ingredients, cooking techniques and how to go grocery shopping for your diet, it will be easier for you to twist and change things in the meal plan. Do not try to change the meal plan for the first 2 weeks. Stick to the meal plan they give you. If you try to change it right at the beginning, you may feel lost or feel terrified in the beginning. So, it is advised to try and introduce new recipes and ideas after you are 2 weeks into the diet.

Drink Lots of Water

Staying hydrated is the key to living a healthy life in general. It is not relevant for only diets, but in general, we should always be drinking enough water to keep ourselves hydrated. Dehydration can bring forth many unwanted diseases. When you are dehydrated, you feel very dizzy, lightheaded, nauseous, and lethargic. You cannot focus on anything well. Urinary infection occurs, which triggers other health issues. Being on a diet, the purpose of drinking water is to help you process the different food you are eating and to help digest it well. Water helps in proper digestion; it helps in extracting bad minerals from our body. Water also gives us a glow on the skin.

Never Skip Breakfast

It is very essential to eat a full breakfast to keep yourself moving actively throughout the day. It gives you a great boost, good metabolism and your digestion starts properly functioning during the day. When you skip breakfast, everything sort of disrupts. Your day starts slow and soon you would feel restless. It is especially important to have a good meal at the beginning of your day in order to be productive for the rest of the day.

If you are terribly busy, try to have your breakfast on the go. Grab a breakfast in a box or a mason jar and have it in the car or in the bus or whatever transport you are using to get to your work. You can also have your breakfast at a healthy restaurant where they serve food that is in sync with your diet.

Eat Protein

Protein is particularly good for the body. It helps your brain function better. Protein can come from both animal and non-animal products. So even if you are a vegetable or vegan, you can still enjoy your protein from plants. Soy, mushroom, legumes, and nuts are a few examples. Eating protein keeps you strong and healthy. Eating protein increases your brain function. On the other hand, if you do not eat enough protein for the day, your entire way would be wasted. You will not be able to focus on anything properly. You would feel dizzy and weak all through the day. If you are a vegetarian, or vegan, you can enjoy avocado, coconut, almond, cashew, soy, and mushroom to get protein.

Eat Super Foods

Most people eat foods which do not necessarily affect them in the best way. Where some foods may enhance some people's energy levels, it may impact others more negatively.

The important thing is to know your food. It may be a good idea to keep a food journal, and if you know that certain foods affect you negatively, one should try to avoid those foods and stick to the healthier options. It is a fact that most people enjoy foods which they should probably not be eating. However, if you wish to eat mindfully and enhance your health and a general sense of wellbeing, then it would be best to eat foods that will precisely do that.

There are also various foods which are classified as superfoods. These would include your lean and purest sources of protein, such as free-range chicken, as well as a variety of fresh fruit, vegetable, and herbs.

Stop Multitasking While You Eat

Multitasking is defined as the simultaneous execution of more than one activity at one time. Though it is a skill that we should master, it often leads to an unproductive activity. The development of our economy leads to a more hectic way of living. Most of us develop the habit of doing one thing while doing another. This is true even when it comes to eating.

Pre-Portion Your Food

Along with meal-prepping and plans, you can pre-portion your food. Let us say you prepared a casserole for Tuesday night's supper. Once the casserole has cooled from cooking, you grab two containers, a larger one and a smaller one. The larger one holds most of the casserole as it is for your family. The smaller container holds your portion, which you can measure out. Then, when you go to warm up the food, you already have your portion separated from everyone else and, because you have already gone through the work of pre-portioning, you're bound to eat that parcel. This likewise helps if you feel somewhat humiliated about administering your food. You should never feel embarrassed about eating healthier, but it is part of our emotions that often cloud us.

Smaller Plates, Taller Glasses

This habit changer ties in a little bit with drinking more water; however, it is a bit different. People tend to fill up their plates with food, so the size of the plate matters. If you have a large plate, you are going to put more food on your plate but, if you have a smaller plate, you will have less food on your plate.

Stay Positive

The secret to succeeding in anything is being positive. When you start something new, always stay positive regarding it. You need to keep a positive mind, an open mind rather. You cannot be anxious, hasty, and restless in a diet. You need to keep calm and do everything that calms you down. Overthinking can lead to being bored and not interested in the diet very soon. The power of positivity is immense. It cannot be compared with anything else. On the other hand, when you start something with a negative mindset, it eventually does not work out. You end up leaving it behind or failing at it because you had doubts right at the beginning. A doubtful mind cannot focus properly, and the best never comes out from a doubtful mind.

Eating mindlessly can cause anyone to eat way too much and this is what happens to most of us. The problem is that when people are eating, they are hardly thinking about what they are doing. Instead, their minds are on other things and this leads them to not be aware of how much they are eating.

Chapter 15: Building the Foundation

It is important to gain insight into the internal and external influences that form you're eating habits, and to cultivate intrinsic motivation partly by interacting with your values. But modifying your behavior will remain discouragingly difficult—not because you are necessarily lazy or self-destructive, but because eating is an ingrained habit that you've been doing for decades.

Researchers have been zeroing in on the neuroscience in recent years, which develops patterns and keeps them in place. Doing an action in a certain way, over time, slowly develops neural pathways within the brain and the behavior is automatic, something we do without thought. This method, known as procedural learning, occurs for routine tasks that most of us learn as children, including brushing our teeth and tying our shoes, and it can occur for eating habits that we've come to follow almost instinctively, whether they're healthy or unhealthy. It is easier to think about any learned behavior as a bundled answer that gets wired into our brains. Some packaged responses include brain parts called reward centers, which make them even more tenacious and complex. Smoking, gambling, drug intake, and consuming high-sugar or high-fat foods fall under this group.

Let us look at a popular one that most of us can recall learning to understand how bundled responses work: driving. If you learned as a teenager, you probably still remember those herky-jerky first attempts that took all your concentration and energy, along with the look of thinly veiled fear on your mother's face, dad, older sibling or driving instructor sitting in the passenger seat. But over time, the different specialized skills needed to drive, steering, accelerating, or braking, changing gears, slowly fused into a smooth, coherent whole. Driving has become automatic, something you do without worrying a great deal about. It is now a packed response after years of practice.

Like driving, eating habits can, over time, be stored as packed responses in our brains. From a health viewpoint, it is worth changing habits to open a Coke every night when you get home or pop chips into your mouth when finishing work tasks. But on a physiological level, eating habits like those are what the brain and

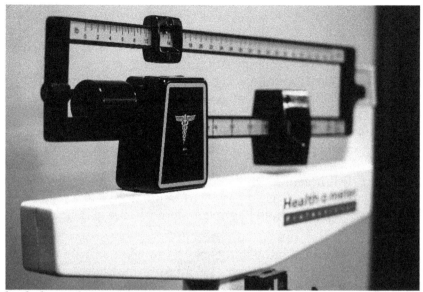

body know how to do.

Packaged eating reactions are more complex than driving or tying your shoes, containing far more chemicals in the body—peptides, hormones, and neurotransmitters. Maybe more important, whatever connections you have developed between eating and emotions can also be packed together: for example, reaching for carbohydrates when you are upset is a popular packed answer. Sometimes, these bundled responses are programmed, incorporated, and stored in our brain physiology. Such connections have probably in the past helped you cope in some way. However, if done too much, the costs outweigh the benefits, and it might be time to develop new relationships.

Rewiring the Brain

The good news is our brains are "soft-wired," not hard-wired. They have neuroplasticity with new neural pathways, which means they can be rewired. That is not a quick or simple process—it takes time, intent and practice. To undo a packaged response such as eating and its associations, you need a method to isolate the package first and foremost.

Enter consciousness. A theory based on everyday practice, consciousness cultivates the mindset and skills required to pick out the individual pieces of a compressed response such as eating—and the resources to improve it.

The skills you will learn here are a type of applied conscientiousness that blends ancient tradition with modern science. The nature of practice—meditation of mindfulness—originates from the teachings of Buddhism. In the 1970s, Jon Kabat-Zinn, Ph.D., developed a program at the University of Massachusetts Medical Center that translated some of those teachings into a secular context, Mindfulness-Based Stress Reduction (MBSR). MBSR has been developed to help people manage stress, pain, and several acute and chronic diseases. MBSR's remarkable popularity it is now being taught at more than 200 health centers and its effects have been confirmed in several studies, has given rise to similar types of applied knowledge, like the mindful eating system you are using.

The heart of the practice of mindfulness is to pay attention consciously, with empathy and curiosity to what you are doing in the present—in both your body and mind. It may not sound like a big deal, but paying attention is the opposite of what we are conditioned to do (to stay unconscious) by both our social culture and our practiced prepared reactions, and the opposite of what most of us do. Practicing mindfulness can disrupt unconscious and reactive behavior—which involves unhealthy eating for many people. You begin to realize the subtle underlying feelings, emotions, and physical sensations that drive the behaviors by practicing mindfulness, and that knowledge is the beginning of improvement.

When you pick apart a packaged answer related to food, you know there are certain facets of automatic actions that you have power over. You discover that what seems like a single event—for example, overeating at lunch—is, in fact, a collection of tiny "micro-events," all connected. You might still be bombarded on your way to your office by the seductive scent of freshly baked muffins at the bakery, but you can pause before you walk in, buy one, and wolf it down; in that pause, you remember and feel the power to make another choice. And paying attention can be creative, easy as it sounds.

However, paying attention is not automatic. It acts, in the form of daily meditation and practice.

Taking the Package Apart: Sensations, Thoughts, and Emotions

Undoing the bundled answers that do not serve you well starts by tuning in to what's going on in your body and mind—specifically, physical stimuli, feelings and emotions.

We're always "in our heads" rather than our bodies, so it provides some valuable knowledge to tun into our bodies. For example, experiencing hunger and fullness signals from your body and the way food tastes will dramatically alter you're eating experience. Or you might find that in the afternoons, after sitting all day at your office, you feel a wave of exhaustion and your shoulders start to ache—and that you prefer to respond by going to the vending machine and buying M&Ms. Noticing stimuli as they arise helps you to respond in a healthier manner, which can avoid the domino effect that contributes to unhealthy eating. For example, if you feel the afternoon tiredness and pain, you can respond by taking a 10-minute walk outside, instead of eating M&Ms.

Identifying your thoughts that sound easy, but for many people it's challenging because we prefer to connect with our thoughts instead of identifying them for what they are: separate mental "events" containing information—information that may or may not be valid and may or may not be helpful. Beliefs—ideas so deeply rooted that we consider them to be real—are especially tenacious. Suppose you are eating a piece of cheesecake, and only "think" that you've done it because you don't have self-control. That so-called information is conviction, not reality. It is important to know that our thoughts can lead us astray. When we think we should be that way, or need other stuff, we sometimes convey patterns or messages absorbed from others or our culture in general. Such convictions are not only always unfounded, they do not serve us well, either. You may ask when you accept a thought or opinion, do I know that to be true? How does the thought make me feel? How do I act on that idea? Take a woman in the dressing room, for example, who actually "knows" that she should be a size 6. Whence comes this "knowledge?" What is it that makes her have the belief? How is she acting upon that belief?

You should practice observing your thoughts during meditation. You will be able to note your emotions in your daily life when you get good at that. And that gives you the chance to analyze them, challenge their validity and alter the actions that motivate those thoughts. In the conventional practice of mindfulness, people learn to observe thoughts as they form—and then the thoughts fade away without requiring a response. If you know in applied awareness whether a thought is false or unhelpful, you can only watch the thought disappear (as in conventional awareness)—or you can alter the thought if it makes you improve your behavior. Suppose your office, for example, is stacked high with paperwork. "My office is something of a mess. I'll never be able to clean it up, "you think—and you'll go to get a snack in response to that thought (even though you're not hungry). When you understand this pattern, you may consciously analyze your thoughts and alter them. The self-defeating thinking, "I'm never going to be able to clean it up," may turn into "I'm going to waste ten minutes sorting the papers on my desk." As for feelings, we are all feeling them but don't really know how to define them or what to do about them. That is partly cultural. Compared to other cultures, our emphasis is very much on problem-solving and doing (instead of being) and thinking rather than feeling. We do not know what feelings can do. So, when feelings are met, they're usually just optimistic ones. The negative ones are messy, uncomfortable, and unreasonable and most of us are learning very little knowledge or skills on how to handle them on our journey to adulthood. Some emotions tend to be shied away from, devalued, and even punished from an early age, such as sadness and rage. Children are told explicitly and implicitly, in certain families and at school, to "be good," not to scream, not to be angry, and not to be afraid.

Under certain conditions, the repression of emotions will mean that they explode in others. We are overcome by the flip side of rejecting feelings, which is also normal. Often people get caught in frustration, snapping at their spouses and kids; or in panic, imagining the most severe cause of unexplained physical symptoms possible. We over-identify with emotions as with thoughts and can't see them for what they are for. Many people respond to emotions—whether they're overwhelming or suppressed.

Mindfulness provides a middle way to deal with feelings, between the extremes of being ignored and swept away by them. As with emotions, the feelings can be felt when holding a wedge of distance—we call this being the Observer. You can see feelings for what they are—and benefit from them when you do so.

You will help improve your eating habits in a variety of ways by being mindful of your inner world—sensations, feelings, and emotions—through mindfulness.

Chapter 16: Overcoming Trauma, Anxiety, and Depression Meditation

Trauma, anxiety, and depression are all difficult things to have to deal with. If you experience one or more of these mental illnesses, then you know that it can be a struggle to get a restful night's sleep.

Anxious thoughts of your past or worries over what might happen tomorrow can really make it hard for you to stay relaxed all throughout the night. Even when you are sleeping, you might have constant nightmares that make it hard for you to feel comfortable in your own bed. In this meditation, we are going to take you through trauma. We are going to make it easier for you to be able to understand how to heal from some of these processes.

What you should know before getting into the meditation is that this is not going to be an instant cure. Mental illness does not go away with the snap of your fingers. It is a constant struggle to find the right mindset to overcome some of your biggest issues. This is a beginner exercise that is going to help unlock some parts of your brain needed to heal. There is a trigger warning for this meditation. We will be talking about wounds and trauma. If at any time your mind seems to wander somewhere dark and you do not understand how to pull yourself from this, feel free to stop and move and do something that distracts you.

Of course, the point of this meditation is going to make sure that you are calm and at peace, but we cannot always help where our minds wander sometimes. If you get stuck in a panic, then remember to simply participate in more breathing exercises.

This meditation will help you heal and find the peace that you need to move on from some of your most challenging issues.

Make sure you are in a comfortable place because towards the end, we are going to encourage you to fall asleep. Keep an open mind and allow your thoughts to flow freely.

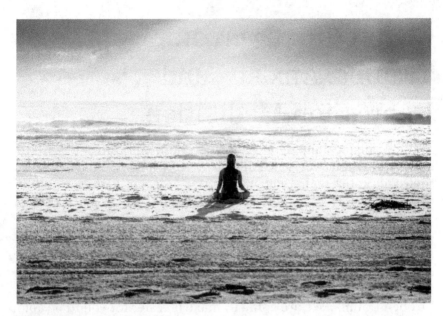

Meditation for Quieting Trauma, Depression, and Anxiety

After you have a physical wound on your body, there are four stages of healing that occur. These stages help to ensure that the wound does not get any worse and that it heals properly so that the rest of your body can still function. When we experience something traumatic or endure consistent depression and anxiety, it can be like a wound on your soul. These mental wounds do not have big ugly scars, like a scrape on your knee or cut on your face might. We must remember, however, that these scars are still there.

These mental wounds are something that we still need to treat properly. In this meditation, we are going to help you understand how you can self-heal so that you can finally get the peace you need at night. Too often we lie awake thinking of the terrible things that we've experienced. How frequently do you find it almost impossible to actually get a restful night's sleep without waking up several times, playing a certain traumatic experience over and over again in your mind? You don't have to be a prisoner of your own experiences anymore. It is time to learn how you can best heal so that these wounds don't hurt.

Begin focusing on your breath right now. This is a great

meditation to do before bed, but anytime that you need to be more relaxed, after dealing with trauma, anxiety, or depression is perfectly fine as well. Ensure that there are no distractions around you. You don't want any people, pets, music, sounds, sights, or anything else to keep you from being able to drift into a healthy and deep sleep. Feel as the air comes in and out of your body. Already, you can notice the way in which your body does what it can to ensure that you're getting taken care of properly. Even without us thinking about it, our bodies are constantly giving us the right things needed to survive.

We breathe, we digest, we live, we pump blood, and our heart beats. All of this continues to happen without us even having to think about it.

We do some of the work, but our body really comes in and does the rest. It knows exactly how to heal itself as well.

Think about this as you continue to breathe in and out. Breathe in through your nose and out through your mouth. This is a great way to keep you focused on your body. This is the method that you can use to ensure that you aren't thinking too hard about all that is negative for you.

Breathe in again, and out again. Breathe in through your nose for five, four, three, two, and one. Breathe out through your mouth for one, two, three, four, and five. Continue to breathe like this throughout the entire meditation.

When you get a cut or a scrape on your body, there are a few things that happen in order to help you heal. The first step that happens after you cut yourself physically is that your body starts to go through hemostasis. This is the way that your body does what it can to stop the bleeding. At first, at this moment, your body is not concerned with healing. Your body is not going to immediately cover up that wound. All that matters are that the blood stops pouring out so that you don't have to lose any more of that.

This is incredibly powerful. This is what we do mentally. As soon as we experience something traumatic, our bodies will try to stop it. It doesn't try to heal. It doesn't try to make sense of what's going on, and it doesn't try to give us a deep explanation to help further establish what we have been through. The only thing that our body does at this moment is trying to make the trauma stop. It does whatever it can to make sure that we don't have to endure this pain anymore. Your body is incredibly powerful like this.

Understand what you might have gone through to make you try and stop the trauma. What experiences did you live through when your body did whatever it could to make this stop?

Did you try to self-sooth using outside sources? Maybe alcohol or drugs were able to stop the constant terror that ran through your mind.

Recognize this and remind yourself that whatever you have experienced is completely normal. This was your way your body tried to heal. We are past the stage now. Now it is time to move on.

After you get a cut and the bleeding has stopped, what occurs is inflammation. This inflammation is your body's way of fighting off any infection. It makes sure that the groundwork is in place for the actual restructuring of your skin to start.

Inflammation can be what occurs in us. This is when we are crying, when we are in pain, when we are screaming from anger, or when we are begging for things to stop. This is the stage that you might have gone through, but you are past this now. Your body was brave enough to pull you from this. You are so strong that you didn't have to deal with this anymore.

Your body did whatever it could to fight off this trauma and prevent it from happening again.

The point of this stage is to start a new growth process. You have moved past the initial fear and shock of what happened, and instead, you're looking for a way to heal. Unfortunately, not all of us understand the way that we are able to heal ourselves. This is when some things can get a little trickier. You are working through this now. You are fighting off this infection from ever coming back and taking over.

Proliferation. This is when the wound can start to close. Finally, it is not a sore spot anymore. This is the part that we need to focus on. You are focused on moving forward now. You understand that this wound is closing. It is finally healing. The skin is connected to itself once again to make sure that nothing can get in and nothing can get out.

Finally, in the stage of healing, your wound can form something new. This is when there might be a scar.

This is when you could be experiencing a reshaping of a physical part of your body. This is what happens to our soul. After we've experienced something traumatic, we never go back to the exact same way that things used to be. Instead, we only move forward and move on to something greater and better in the end.

Some people's wounds might heal incorrectly. They might let it become scar tissue on their soul, stopping another thing from functioning properly. You are not going to let this happen. You are healing now. You are feeling that wound finally close up. You don't have to let the feelings and emotions that you had at the time pour out anymore.

You're not closing things up so that you never deal with it again. You are simply closing it up because you are stronger and better now. You are moving past these challenging emotions. No longer do you have the challenging thoughts and feelings that used to pop up so frequently in the past.

The thing about scar tissue is that it will never be the same. Some scars will heal perfectly normally, and we don't even have to think about it. Then, there are plenty of other scars that can leave huge marks that can't be looked past. Eventually you'll get used to it. It is a part of you now, and this does not have to be so ugly. We don't have to consider scars as something scary or grotesque. They are simply another marking on our bodies. How many marks do you have simply from not even realizing that they are there?

Maybe there's a freckle on your cheek or a little cut on your arm from when you were a child and fell off your bike. Maybe you have some acne from when you were a teenager, struggling with the constant constellation of pimples across your face. Perhaps you can't grow hair on a certain patch on your body because of the scar. Maybe there's a big ugly lump on your leg that you hate to look at.

Whatever these are, we don't have to be afraid of them just like you don't have to fear the scar that is on your soul. You are moving on and past this now into a happier and healthier place. This scar is part of what makes you beautiful. Think of all the markings on a physical object that you see. Maybe you pull a little penny out of your change purse and notice all the small markings on this.

Chapter 17: Lose Weight Fast and Naturally

Numerous individuals are uncertain about how to lose weight securely and normally. It does not support that multiple sites and notices, especially those having a place with companies that sell diet drugs or other weight-loss products, promote misinformation about losing weight.

As indicated by 2014 research, a great many people who look for tips on the most proficient method to get thinner will go over false or deluding information on weight reduction.

"Fad" diets and exercise regimens can, at times, be hazardous as they can keep individuals from meeting their nourishing needs.

As indicated by the Centers for Disease Control and Prevention, the most secure measure of weight to lose every week is somewhere in the range of 1 and 2 pounds. The individuals who suffer substantially more every week or attempt craze diets or projects are significantly more prone to recover weight.

21. Keeping Refreshing Bites at Home and In the Workplace

Individuals frequently pick to eat nourishments that are helpful, so it is ideal to abstain from keeping prepackaged tidbits and confections close by.

One investigation found that individuals who kept unhealthful nourishment at home thought that it was increasingly hard to keep up or lose weight.

Keeping healthty snacks at home and work can enable an individual to meet their nourishing needs and maintain a strategic distance from an abundance of sugar and salt. Great snack choices include:

- Nuts with no added salt or sugar
- Natural products
- Prechopped vegetables
- Low-fat yoghurts
- Dried seaweed

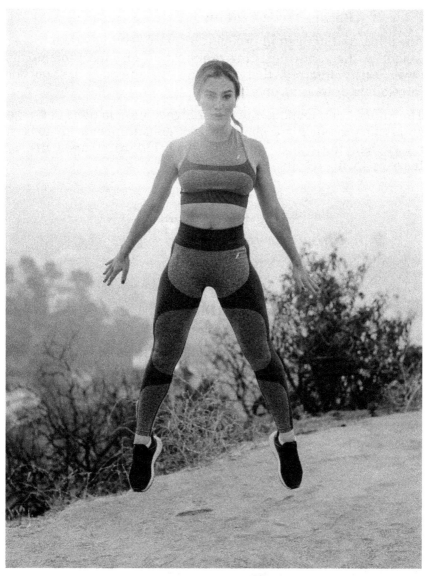

22. Removing Processed Foods

Processed foods are high in sodium, fat, calories, and sugar. They frequently contain fewer supplements than entire nourishments.

As indicated by a primer research study, processed foods are substantially more likely than different food sources to prompt addictive eating practices, which will, in general outcome in individuals indulging.

23. Eating More Protein

An eating routine high in protein can enable an individual to lose weight. A diagram of existing examination on high protein eats fewer carbs inferred that they are an effective system for forestalling or treating obesity.

The information demonstrated that higher-protein diets of 25–30 grams of protein for each feast gave enhancements in hunger, bodyweight the board, cardiometabolic hazard components, or these wellbeing results.

- Fish
- Beans, peas, and lentils
- White poultry
- Low-fat cottage cheese
- Tofu

24. Stopping Included Sugar

Sugar is not in every case simple to maintain a strategic distance from; however, disposing of handled nourishments is a positive initial step to take.

As per the National Cancer Institute, men matured 19 years and more established devour a normal of more than 19 teaspoons of included sugar a day. Ladies in a similar age bunch eat more than 14 teaspoons of added sugar a day.

A significant part of the sugar that individuals devour originates from fructose, which the liver separates and transforms into fat. After the liver converts the sugar into fat, it discharges these fat cells into the blood, which can prompt weight gain.

25. Drinking Black Coffee

Coffee may have some constructive wellbeing impacts if an individual forgoes, including sugar and fat. The writers of a survey article saw that coffee improved the body's processing of carbohydrates and fats.

A like look at featured a relationship between coffee utilization and a lower danger of diabetes and liver disease.

26. Remaining Hydrated

Water is the best liquid that an individual can drink for the day. It contains no calories and gives an abundance of health benefits.

At the point when an individual drinks water for the day, the water helps increment their digestion. Drinking water before a feast can likewise help decrease the sum that they eat.

At long last, if individuals supplant sweet refreshments with water, this will help decrease all outnumber of calories that they devour for the day.

27. Keeping Away from The Calories in Beverages

Soft drinks, natural product squeezes, and sports and caffeinated drinks regularly contain abundant sugar, which can prompt weight increase and make it progressively hard for an individual to get in shape.

Other high-calorie drinks incorporate liquor and strength espressos, like lattes, which contain milk and sugar.

Individuals can have a go at supplanting, at any rate, one of these drinks every day with water, shining water with lemon, or an herbal tea.

28. Avoiding Refined Carbohydrates

Proof in The American Journal of Clinical Nutrition recommends that refined sugars might be more harmful to the body's digestion than saturated fats.

Considering the convergence of sugar from refined starches, the liver will make and discharge fat into the circulatory system.

To diminish weight and keep it off, an individual can eat entire grains.

Refined or simple carbohydrates incorporate the accompanying nourishments:

- White rice
- White bread
- White flour
- Candies
- Numerous sorts of cereal
- Included sugars
- Numerous sorts of pasta

Rice, bread, and pasta are, for the most part, accessible in entire grain varieties, which can help weight reduction and help shield the body from disease.

29. Fasting in Cycles

Fasting for short periods may enable an individual to get more fit. As per a recent report, irregular fasting or substitute day fasting can allow an individual to get in shape and keep up their weight reduction.

However, not every person should quick. Fasting can be dangerous for kids, creating adolescents, pregnant ladies, older individuals, and individuals with hidden wellbeing conditions.

30. Counting Calories and Keeping A Nourishment Diary

Counting calories can be a viable method to abstain from gorging. By tallying calories, an individual will know about precisely the amount they are devouring. This mindfulness can assist them with removing superfluous calories and settle on better dietary decisions.

A nourishment diary can enable an individual to consider what and the amount they are devouring each day. By doing this, they can likewise guarantee that they are getting enough of each stimulating nutrition type, for example, vegetables and proteins.

31. Brushing Teeth Between Dinners or Prior at Night

Notwithstanding improving dental cleanliness, brushing the teeth can help lessen the impulse to nibble between dinners.

If an individual who regularly snacks around evening time brushes their teeth prior at night, they may feel less enticed to eat extra snacks.

32. Eating More Fruits and Vegetables

An eating routine wealthy in products of the soil can enable an individual to get more fit and keep up their weight reduction.

The author of an orderly survey supports this case, expressing that advancing an expansion in products of the soil utilization is probably not going to cause any weight increase, even without instructing individuals to diminish their use regarding different nourishments.

33. Lessening Carbohydrate Consumption

Diets low in basic starches can enable an individual to reduce their weight by constraining the measure of added sugar that they eat.

Restorative low carbohydrate abstains from food center around expending entire sugars, high fats, fiber, and lean proteins. Rather than restricting all sugars for a brief period, this ought to be a reasonable, long haul dietary alteration.

34. Eating More Fiber

Fiber offers a few potential advantages to an individual hoping to get thinner. Research in Nutrition expresses that an expansion in fiber utilization can enable an individual to feel fuller more rapidly.

Furthermore, fiber helps weight reduction by advancing absorption and adjusting the microorganisms in the gut.

35. Expanding Traditional Cardiovascular and Resistance Training

Numerous individuals do not practice regularly and may likewise have inactive occupations. It is critical to incorporate both cardiovascular (cardio) work out, for example, running or strolling, and opposition preparing in a regular exercise program.

Cardio enables the body to consume calories rapidly while obstruction preparing manufactures fit bulk. Bulk can assist individuals with consuming more calories very still.

Furthermore, explore has discovered that individuals who take an interest in high-intensity interval training (HIIT) can lose more weight and see more prominent enhancements in their cardiovascular wellbeing than individuals who are utilizing other mainstream strategies for weight reduction.

36. Devouring Whey Protein

Individuals who use whey protein may expand their slender bulk while diminishing muscle versus fat, which can help with weight reduction.

Research from 2014 found that whey protein, in the mix with practice or a weight reduction diet, may help diminish body weight and muscle to fat ratio.

37. Eating Slowly

Eating slowly can enable an individual to decrease all outnumber of calories that they expend in one sitting. The purpose behind this is it can require some investment to understand that the stomach is full.

One examination showed that eating rapidly relates to corpulence. While the investigation couldn't prescribe mediations to enable an individual to eat all the more gradually, the outcomes do propose that eating nourishment at a slower pace can help decrease calorie consumption.

Biting nourishment completely and eating at a table with others may enable an individual to back off while eating.

38.Including Chili

Adding spice to nourishments may enable an individual to get more fit. Capsaicin is a compound that is normally present in flavors, for example, bean stew powder, and may have constructive outcomes.

For instance, inquire about demonstrates that capsaicin can assist ignite with fatting and increment digestion, yet at low rates.

39.Getting More Sleep

There is a link between corpulence and an absence of value rest. The research proposes that getting adequate rest can add to weight loss. The researchers found that ladies who depicted their rest quality as poor or reasonable were more averse to effectively get in shape than the individuals who detailed their rest quality as being generally excellent.

40.   Utilizing a Smaller Plate

Utilizing smaller plates could have a positive mental impact. Individuals will, in general, fill their plate, so lessening the size of the plate may help decrease the measure of nourishment that an individual eats in one sitting. A 2015 systematic reassessment inferred that diminishing plate size could affect partition control and vitality utilization, yet it was hazy whether this was material over the full scope of bit sizes. Individuals hoping to get in shape securely and normally should concentrate on making a perpetual way of life changes instead of embracing brief measures.

Individuals must concentrate on making changes that they can keep up. Now and again, an individual may want to execute changes steadily or take a stab at presenting each in turn.

Chapter 18: Learning to Avoid Temptations and Triggers

While telling a person to adopt the traits of the mentally strong is a good way to develop mental toughness, it may not always be enough. In a way, it's a bit like telling a person that in order to be healthy you need to eat right, exercise, and get plenty of rest. Such advice is good and even correct, however, it lacks a certain specificity that can leave a person feeling unsure of exactly what to do. Fortunately, there are several practices that can create a clear plan of how to achieve mental toughness. These practices are like the actual recipes and exercises needed in order to eat right and get plenty of exercises. By adopting these practices into your daily routine, you will begin to develop mental toughness in everything you do and, in every environment, you find yourself in.

Keep Your Emotions in Check

The most important thing you can do in the quest for developing mental toughness is to keep your emotions in check. People who fail to take control of their emotions allow their emotions to control them. More often than not, this takes the form of people who are driven by rage, fear, or both. Whenever a person allows their emotions to control them, they allow their emotions to control their decisions, words, and actions. However, when you keep your emotions in check, you take control of your decisions, words, and actions, thereby taking control of your life overall.

In order to keep your emotions in check you have to learn to allow your emotions to subside before reacting to a situation. Therefore, instead of speaking when you are angry, or making a decision when you are frustrated, take a few minutes to allow your emotions to settle down. Take a moment to simply sit down, breathe deeply, and allow your energies to restore balance. Only when you feel calm and in control should you make your decision, speak your mind, or take any action.

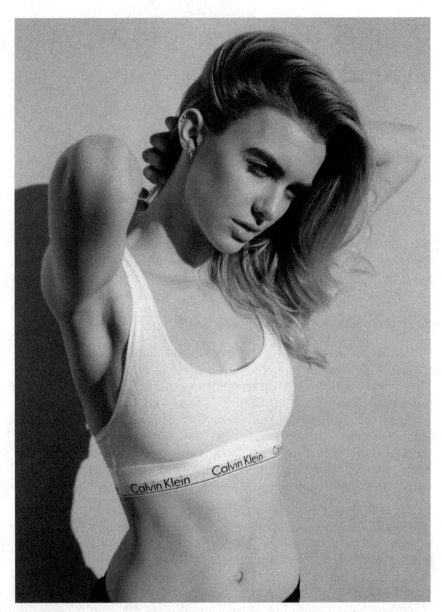

Practice Detachment

Another critical element for mental toughness is what is known as detachment. This is when you remove yourself emotionally from the particular situation that is going on around you. Even if the situation affects you directly, remaining detached is a very positive thing. The biggest benefit of detachment is that it prevents an emotional response to the situation at hand. This is particularly helpful when things are not going according to plan.

Practicing detachment requires a great deal of effort at first. After all, most people are programmed to feel emotionally attached to the events going on around them at any given time. One of the best ways to practice detachment is to tell yourself that the situation isn't permanent. What causes a person to feel fear and frustration when faced with a negative situation is that they feel the situation is permanent. When you realize that even the worst events are temporary, you avoid the negative emotional response they can create.

Another way to become detached is to determine the reason you feel attached to the situation in the first place. In the case that someone is saying or doing something to hurt your feelings, understand that their words and actions are a reflection of them, not you. As long as you don't feed into their negativity you won't experience the pain they are trying to cause. This is true for anything you experience. By not feeding a negative situation or event with negative emotions, you prevent that situation from connecting to you. This allows you to exist within a negative event without being affected by it.

Accept What Is Beyond Your Control

Acceptance is one of the cornerstones of mental toughness. This can take the form of accepting yourself for who you are and accepting others for who they are, but it can also take the form of accepting what is beyond your control. When you learn to accept the things you can't change, you rewrite how your mind reacts to every situation you encounter. The fact of the matter is that the majority of stress and anxiety felt by the average person is the result of not being able to change certain things. Once you learn to accept those things you can't change, you eliminate all of that harmful stress and anxiety permanently.

While accepting what is beyond your control will take a little practice, it is actually quite easy in nature. The trick is to simply ask yourself if you can do anything at all to change the situation at hand. If the answer is 'no,' simply let it go. Rather than wasting time and energy fretting about what you can't control, adopt the mantra "It is what it is." This might seem careless at first, but after a while you will realize that it is a true sign of mental strength. By accepting what is beyond your control, you conserve your energy, thoughts, and time for those things you can affect, thereby making your efforts more effective and worthwhile.

Always Be Prepared

Another way to build mental toughness is to always be prepared. If you allow life to take you from one event to another, you will feel lost, uncertain, and unprepared for the experiences you encounter. However, when you take the time to prepare yourself for what lies ahead, you will develop a sense of being in control of your situation at all times. There are two ways to be prepared, and they are equally important for developing mental toughness.

The first way to be prepared is to prepare your mind at the beginning of each and every day. This takes the form of you taking time in the morning to focus your mind on who you are, what you are capable of, and your outlook on life in general. Whether you refer to this time as mediation, contemplation, or daily affirmations, the basic principle is the same. You simply focus your mind on what you believe and the qualities you aspire to. This will keep you grounded in your ideals throughout the day, helping you to make the right choices regardless of what life throws your way.

The second way to always be prepared is to take the time to prepare yourself for the situation at hand. If you have to give a presentation, make sure to give yourself plenty of time to prepare for it. Go over the information you want to present, choose the materials you want to use, and even take the time to make sure you have the exact clothes you want to wear. When you go into a situation fully prepared, you increase your self-confidence, giving you an added edge. Additionally, you will eliminate the stress and anxiety that results from feeling unprepared.

Take the Time to Embrace Success

One of the problems many negatively minded people experience is that they never take the time to appreciate success when it comes to their way. Sometimes they are too afraid of jinxing that success to actually recognize it. Most of the time, however, they are unable to embrace success because their mindset is simply too negative for such a positive action. Mentally strong people, by contrast, always take the time to embrace the successes that come their way. This serves to build their sense of confidence as well as their feeling of satisfaction with how things are going.

Following time, you experience a success of any kind, make sure you take a moment to recognize it. You can make an external statement, such as going out for drinks, treating yourself to a nice lunch, or some similar expression of gratitude. Alternatively, you can simply take a quiet moment to reflect on the success and all the effort that went into making it happen. There is no right or wrong way to embrace success, you just need to find a way that works for you. The trick to embracing success is in not letting it go to your head. Rather than praising your efforts or actions, appreciate the fact that things went well. Also, be sure to appreciate those whose help contributed to your success.

Be happy with what you have

Contentment is another element that is critical for mental toughness. In order to develop contentment, you have to learn how to be happy with what you have. This doesn't mean that you eliminate ambition or the desire to achieve greater success, rather it means that you show gratitude for the positives that currently exist. After all, the only way you will be able to truly appreciate the fulfillment of your dreams is if you can first appreciate your life the way it is. One example of this is learning to appreciate your job. This is true whether you like your job or not. Even if you hate your job and desperately want to find another one, always take the time to appreciate the fact that you have a job in the first place. The fact is that you could be jobless, which would create all sorts of problems in your life. So, even if you hate your job, learn to appreciate it for what it is. This goes for everything in your life. No matter how good or bad a thing is, always appreciate having it before striving to make a change.

Be Happy with Who You Are

In addition to appreciating what you have, you should always be happy with who you are. Again, this doesn't mean that you should settle for who you are and not try to improve your life, rather it means that you should learn to appreciate who you are at every moment. There will always be issues that you want to fix in your life, and things you know you could do better. The problem is that if you focus on the things that are wrong, you will always see yourself in a negative light. However, when you learn to appreciate the good parts of your personality, you can pursue self-improvement with a sense of pride, hope, and optimism for who you will become as you begin to fulfill your true potential.

Chapter 19: Weight Loss Through Self Hypnosis

Hypnosis can stop those anomalous wants and noon sneaking into the kitchen. Overall, let us delve into the genuine meaning of hypnosis to build up realities in that impact. Hypnosis is a psychological state where you are in a stupor, where you are dependent upon recommendations, self-proposal, or autosuggestions. In hypnotherapy meetings, you are in hypnotic acceptance where you are increasingly responsive to new thoughts and orders since the mind is in an open state.

Is it extremely compelling? How can it work? Before whatever else, this is not enchantment. In contrast to the prevalent view, it cannot mysteriously reboot, reset, or reconstruct the human mind to accomplish results. It is a progression of outrageous fixation followed by unwinding and center that actuates the mind to redesign its eating propensities and hold them reliably. As per anderbilt edu, considers indicating weight loss because of hypnosis alone are very few and experience the ill effects of methodological issues. Some individuals suffered hypnosis for weight loss, and following 12 weeks, the damage a normal of 10.2lbs. The outcomes were promising and fascinating to the media, yet the benchmark group was little, and we cannot sum up the finding that it will be compelling to everybody.

The center of the hypnosis treatment for weight loss is to reinvent or change an individual's conduct towards nourishment, diet, and different variables that trigger weight loss. For instance, if one individual is inclined to binges on account of emotional eating, hypnosis can propose new responses. At the point when looked by a terrible day or nearly at the highest point of emotional eating, one can suggest that as opposed to venting out on dessert, one can go to the rec center and exercise.

Hypnosis results pass on that it is critical to realize that social change in relationship with weight the executives are unquestionably more essential and viable than hypnosis alone. You can ask your therapist or a hypnosis expert regarding this, yet before you submit on anything, talk with your doctor first. It is unequivocally recommended that you ensure the impacts of a changed eating example to your wellbeing. Here and there, eating designs are reactions to some hidden neurotic as well as dietary infirmities, for example, diabetes. For the individuals who have nourishment irregularity, be additional careful in putting your mind under hypnosis. Your wellbeing emphatically relies upon how and what you eat. Changing them implies putting your wellbeing needs undermined.

Traditionally, the main way individuals can accomplish weight loss is through sweating it off in the exercise center and essentially starving themselves in a diet that causes them to feel denied and testy. Today a lot of options and one of a kind strategy has been found to support dieters, and weight loss through hypnosis is one of these ways. Utilizing hypnosis to help accomplish weight loss works under the rule that weight loss starts with the mind. You can utilize your mind to control all that you do, and when allurements come to keep you off your track, your first and most grounded weapon to battle this enticement is your mind. Regardless of whether you inevitably win the weight loss fight through dieting and working out, having a prepared and taught mind could spell the distinction among progress and disappointment.

Weight loss through hypnosis considers the way that the mind is your most grounded weapon with regards to getting more fit, and this is the thing that it taps. Hypnosis is the point at which an individual is brought under a modified condition of cognizance, and it has been utilized for social examinations and purposes. A few people are recommending that a trance specialist can be tapped to spellbind the individual who is attempting to lose the weight and adjust key practices that will enable that individual to lose the weight. It is not necessarily the case that hypnosis will work essentially all alone. Despite what might be expected, weight loss through hypnosis is simply utilized as a device to make the ordinary techniques considerably progressively powerful.

Hypnosis along these lines is only a path for individuals to get an adjusted mental cognizance concerning how they see their excursion. This is just powerful whenever taken together with a compelling project. By the day's end, shedding pounds is tied in with practicing normally and satisfactorily, just as controlling the sort and the measure of nourishment that you eat. These dietary limitations and exercise necessities need a ton of control and resolution, and this is the place hypnosis comes in. You cannot win your fight with overabundance weight without enough resolution, because the fight starts with the mind. Self-discipline influences how solid you are in observing your weight loss program through to the end.

What Does Weight Loss Through Hypnosis Take?

Getting More Fit Is an Included Procedure

A lot should be tended to and changed to get more fit. No incredible new data for you there. In any case, did you realize that by utilizing weight loss through hypnosis, you could make that procedure simpler and increasingly pleasurable? You can make it a programmed foolish procedure that, when you remain with it, will bring you down to a significantly more alluring and attractive weight. In the following couple of seconds, I will give you one of the manners in which you can do this.

You have presumably been on diets previously and battled to keep up a prohibitive diet. Furthermore, what occurs? At the point when somebody, even you, reveals to you that you cannot eat a specific nourishment, that nourishment turns out to be much progressively attractive. You begin to want that specific nourishment, not because you need it, but since you cannot have it. These prohibitive projects additionally have another drawback. When you confine your nourishment admission to too scarcely any calories, your body, through an endurance instrument, thinks there is starvation and begins to hinder your digestion from moderating your vitality stores—the exact inverse of what you need to occur if you are attempting to get in shape. So prohibitive diets do not work. It is simply that basic.

Furthermore, if you've at any point been on a tight eating routine, you most likely saw this as obvious. You restored all the weight when you quit eating in that prohibitive way. Things can be distinctive when you use weight loss through hypnosis.

Things being what they are, by what method can weight loss through hypnosis improve this procedure?

At the point when you are entranced, something that an accomplished and very much prepared subliminal specialist will have the option to do is to change your reaction to nourishment and eating. We are brought into the world with the best possible conduct toward nourishment that we need to have. That conduct is to eat when hungry and stop when full. Have you, at any point, see how a newborn child eats? A baby eats until it is full and afterward stops. It lets out the areola and will eat because it need not bother with the nourishment any longer. It has provided itself with the fundamental supplements it requires to deal with its requirements for the following couple of hours.

Recapturing the Apparatuses Given You During Childbirth

You were brought into the world with that equivalent capacity. A very much prepared trance inducer can make the states that are essential for you to make changes in your reactions and responses to foods... even the contemplations of nourishment. Furthermore, by doing only this straightforward procedure, you begin to see nourishment and eating unexpectedly. You are never again constrained by nourishment. You are happy with a limited quantity of nourishment. You recover power over the straightforward undertaking of providing supplements to your body, and that feels better.

This is only one of the techniques that are utilized in helping you recapture command over nourishment and shed pounds utilizing hypnosis for weight loss.

So, if you need to encounter weight loss through hypnosis to assist you with losing weight, something you need is to make the state where nourishment is simply one more item that we use to supply life, such as breathing and drinking water. You can move nourishment out of your awareness with the goal that it is the thing that it was proposed to be, a characteristic component like air, utilized for supporting life.

Weight Loss through Hypnosis - Hype or Not

Consistently, you are shelled with new items out in the market, guaranteeing that such and such an item can assist you with shedding 10 pounds in about fourteen days or assist you with being a skinnier individual in only one month. Have you ever caught wind of weight loss through hypnosis? There are a lot of surveys been done about this procedure. Some surveys offered go-ahead for hypnosis, and there are some who scrutinized its validity and the fundamental motivation behind why an individual can shed pounds through it.

Is it enchantment, or is it a logical truth? Weight loss through hypnosis may sound persuading; however, accomplishes it truly work? Like some other weight loss program or item, everything relies upon the distinct individual. One may work for you and not for your companion. This new thought of hypnosis comparable to weight loss has been given accentuation while contemplates have uncovered that the individuals who have experienced the procedure without a doubt lose the weight and even kept it up after some time.

The mystery? Your mind. The mind is ground-breaking to such an extent that it very well may be the way to helping you lose those pounds you constantly needed to lose. You can discover CDs that contain a few projects that can help you in molding your brain and oversee your life.

You can get data on the how-to and the things expected to make weight loss through hypnosis like how to supplant undesirable propensities with sound ones, how to check your longings and be in charge rather than your weight controlling your life. These CDs contain portrayal and guidelines. It resembles somebody is conversing with you, in a quieting voice while inspiring you to carry on with a solid way of life while getting in shape. It resembles having a companion who can help you when you are at an intersection in your life.

The mind can do it can wreck or improve your life. Everything happens directly inside your mind. At the point when you know how to control your desires, inspire yourself, or be taught in arriving at your objective, then certainly you will have the body you constantly needed for the long haul.

Chapter 20: Daily Guided Meditation Techniques

3 Minutes Guided Meditation

Sit comfortably in a cross-legged posture

If you are not comfortable sitting in a cross-legged posture, position yourself on a chair

Keep your back straight

You can use a backrest but not a headrest

Close your eyes comfortably

Start breathing normally

Breathe in slowly

Let the air enter through your nostrils

Feel the warmth of the air as it enters

Fill your lungs with the air

Feel it entering your abdomen

Hold your breath for a few moments

Now, release the breath slowly through your mouth

Breathe in slowly

Hold your breath

Breathe out

Thoughts may start entering your mind

Pay no attention to them

If your attention is getting diverted

Simply observe the thoughts but don't get involved

Focus on your breathing

Breathe in

Breathe out

If you are getting distracted

Breathe in and count backward from 4

4...3...2...1

Hold your breath to the count backward from 4

4...3...2...1

Release your breath slowly backward to the count of 7

7...6...5...4...3...2...1

Repeat this process 3 times

Breathe in and count backward from 4

4...3...2...1

Hold your breath to the count backward from 4

4...3...2...1

Release your breath slowly backward to the count of 7

7...6...5...4...3...2...1

Every exhalation takes away stress and negativity

Breathe in and count backward from 4

4...3...2...1

Hold your breath to the count backward from 4

4...3...2...1

Release your breath slowly backward to the count of 7

7...6...5...4...3...2...1

You are feeling good, there is nothing disturbing you

Breathe in and count backward from 4

4...3...2...1

Hold your breath to the count backward from 4

4...3...2...1

Release your breath slowly backward to the count of 7

7...6...5...4...3...2...1

You are calm and relaxed now

Your mind would get settled and the thoughts wouldn't disturb you

Now start breathing normally and become aware of your surroundings

Open your eyes gently

5 Minutes Guided Meditation

Sit comfortably in a cross-legged posture

If you are not comfortable sitting in a cross-legged posture, position yourself on a chair

Keep your back straight

You can use a backrest but not a headrest

Close your eyes comfortably

Start breathing normally

Breathe in slowly

Let the air enter through your nostrils

Feel the warmth of the air as it enters

Fill your lungs with the air

Feel it entering your abdomen

Hold your breath for a few moments

Now, release the breath slowly through your mouth

Breathe in slowly

Hold your breath

Breathe out

Thoughts may start entering your mind

Pay no attention to them

If your attention is getting diverted

Simply observe the thoughts but do not get involved

Focus on your breathing

Breathe in

Breathe out

If you are getting distracted

Breathe in and count backward from 4

4...3...2...1

Hold your breath to the count backward from 4

4...3...2...1

Release your breath slowly backward to the count of 7

7...6...5...4...3...2...1

Your mind became calm

Your body release any tension

Repeat this process 3 times

Breathe in and count backward from 4

4...3...2...1

Hold your breath to the count backward from 4

4...3...2...1

Release your breath slowly backward to the count of 7

7...6...5...4...3...2...1

Breathe in and count backward from 4

4...3...2...1

Hold your breath to the count backward from 4

4...3...2...1

Release your breath slowly backward to the count of 7

7...6...5...4...3...2...1

Breathe in and count backward from 4

4...3...2...1

Hold your breath to the count backward from 4

4...3...2...1

Release your breath slowly backward to the count of 7

7...6...5...4...3...2...1

Now, look at the thoughts in your mind

Become aware of those thoughts

Simply observe them from a distance

Do not take part in them

Do not judge these thoughts

Simply observe the kind of thoughts originating in your mind

They do not concern you now

You do not need to react to these thoughts

Simply become aware of them

Once you become fully aware of these thoughts, they will stop affecting you

Do not run from these thoughts

Accept and embrace them

Bring your attention to your bringing

It is the most important thing now

Breathe in

Hold your breath

Breathe out

Breathe in

Hold your breath

Breathe out

You are very calm and aware

Breathe in

Hold your breath

Breathe out

You are feeling calm and relaxed now

There is no rush

No anxiety

No stress

No anger

No judgment

There is complete calm

Now start breathing normally and become aware of your surroundings

Open your eyes gently

7 Minute Guided Meditation

Take your position at the place of your meditation

Be seated

Sit in a completely relaxed manner

Do not do anything immediately

Ground yourself first

Just sit completely relaxed for a few minutes

Get into a comfortable position

Keep your back straight

Ensure that your shoulders are also straight

Your back and neck should be in a straight line

Now, close your eyes

Lean slightly forward and then backward

Lean-to your left side and then to your right

Now, bring yourself to the center and find the best and most comfortable position

Feel your head positioned on your neck

Raise your chin slightly upwards

This will help you in placing your focus between your eyebrows

Try to feel your whole body

Notice if there is tension anywhere

If you feel any part tense, release the tension

Adjust your body to release the pressure

Now start breathing normally

Inhale through your nose

Exhale through your mouth

Take short inhalations

Hold your breath for a few seconds

Exhale through your mouth longer

Breathe in

Breathe out

Breathe in

Breathe out

Breathe in

Breathe out

Now, focus on the air you are breathing

Feel the warmth of this air

Trace the path taken by the air in your body

Watch it entering your lungs

Feel the expansion of your chest

Feel your stomach getting inflated

Hold your breath for a few seconds now

Count till 4

1....2....3....4

Now, exhale slowly through your mouth

Exhale for the count of 7

1....2....3....4......5....6....7

Again, repeat the process

Inhale to the count of 4

1....2....3....4

Feel it entering your body

Hold your breath for a few seconds now

Count till 4

1....2....3....4

Now, exhale slowly through your mouth

Exhale for the count of 7

1....2....3....4......5....6....7

You are feeling relaxed now

As you exhale you drive away from the negative thoughts and emotions

You are breathing in positivity

Smile as you breathe every time

Feel relaxed as you exhale

This relaxation is natural

It is the natural state of your body

Your body is designed to remain in a relaxed state

You are working to bring it into its natural state

Do not be bothered by your thoughts and emotions

Thoughts will come into your mind

There is no need to worry about them

The harder you will try to push them

The more aggressive they will get

You must embrace and accept them

You should not get affected by them

You should not judge them

Simply observe them from a distance

Like someone observes the traffic on the road standing in the balcony

The traffic is not a problem for that person

It is still there

But that person is not stuck in it

For his, those are some cars standing behind each other

There is no inconvenience

In the same way, these thoughts should also not be a problem for you

They should invoke no reaction

You are not involved in them actively

You are simply observing their creation and futility

You are not interested in them

They cannot affect you

You are getting bored with them

Bring back your focus to your breathing

Inhale slowly

Watch your chest rise as the air fills your lungs

Watch your stomach inflate as air enters it

Hold your breath for a few seconds

Pressure is building

Now slowly exhale

All the pressure inside you will go away with the breath

You are feeling light with every exhale

You are feeling great

This is an amazingly liberating feeling

Repeat the process again

Breathe in

Hold the breath

Exhale slowly

Now your mind is getting clear

You are feeling relaxed

There are no worries

There is no stress

You are feeling light

Focus once again on your breath

Inhale deeply

Let the air enter your body freely

Let it take its own course

Simply follow the path the air takes

Hold it for a few seconds

Now observe the remaining stress going out with the breath

Now start breathing normally

Stabilize your breathing

Let it return to its normal rate

Remain seated with your eyes closed

Try to feel your surrounding

You are feeling very relaxed now

You can open your eyes.

Chapter 21: Background Information for Weight Loss

Understand Your Habits

You may find yourself developing some habits without knowing. The same applies to create excellent health practice. Your daily practices and choices explain your current conditions. Stop complaining; do focus on your habits, remember your preferences will define who you will be. Albert Einstein goes on to say, "we cannot solve our problems with the same thinking we used when we created them." Step out of your bubble a given structure for the desired outcome. Really the hardest part is starting, and you've already done that, and it will only get more accessible and more natural the more you participate and the more you take an active role in this journey.

Consider habits development as elaborated in the story of a Miller and a camel on a winter day. It was freezing outside, and while the miller was asleep, he was awakened by some noise on the door. Upon opening his eyes, he heard the voice of a camel complaining that it was cold outside and was requesting to warm his nose inside. Miller agreed that he was only to insert the nozzle. A little later, the camel put his forehead then the neck, then other parts of the body than the whole-body bit by bit until he started destroying things inside. He started walking in the house, stumbling on anything on its way. When the miller ordered the camel to move out, the came boasted that he was comfortable inside and would not leave. The camel went further to tell the miller that he could leave at his pleasure. The same goes for a habit that comes knocking about and taking over.

Maybe you started out smoking your first cigarette, thinking it was disgusting, and then years go by, and you have a nasty habit. Well, bad habits can sneak in, but the same philosophy can apply to ethical practices. Just take it bit by bit and step by step, and before you know it, you have healthy habits in your life. There are so many challenges to healthy eating. You have to be willing to have an open mind and reset your thinking on food.

It is cheaper to develop new habits; effort is the primary requirement, but not that much. When you have trained yourself new patterns, train on it every day for some time, after which it will be automatic.

We can relate that situation to a football club Coach who engages in various rigorous training with his players while awaiting the actual match. They practice new skills and moves. When match day arrives, the coach sits with the substitutes while watching the players playing from the line. Players play as per the learned skills and moves. Apply the required effort to actualize your goal.

While storying with your workmates, tell them how you drink 3 to for four glasses of water every day, the same as tea. That looks strict. In heart, you know how your consumption of water and team is reduced while at home. This is self-discipline. Self-discipline calls for the establishment of strong foundations. Efforts adopted is less.

Apply Core solutions

Recognize and face the challenges of healthy eating and develop new habits. Like a logger trying to clear a log, identify the critical side of each situation. The well-experienced logger will try to identify essential joints by climbing up then do the clearing. A less experienced logger would start by the edge. Both methods produce expected results, but one way saves more time and uses less energy than the other. All our problems have strategic points. How about when we identify critical logs to healthy eating and offer some solutions. First, log jam. How you were brought up. You may have been forced as a child to eat vegetables and see it as something undesirable, and you built a perception that plants don't taste good. Another log jam is stress. So much pressure.

We live in a world full of pressure where time matters in all our undertakings, troubled life, and our body pay most of the price. You have many choices to pick from. If you are a lover of fast food, you need to stop. Fast foods are addictive, and we highly depend on them due to the positive attitude we have towards them. We are obsessed with them such that we cannot live a day without consuming them. When you eat something wrong for you and you say, you don't care. Your thoughts and focus are totally on how delicious and enjoyable it is to be eating the food that you're eating, regardless of how unhealthy it is, and then you have guilt about how those pounds are going on rather than coming off.

Such thoughts occur even when taking tasty food. We may find ourselves eating some food which in reality we know are very dangerous to our health. Chip is a prime example. An individual from a diet class may feel hungry on her way back home and decide to a branch by a fast food joint for some plates of chips. Despite several cautions on the dangers of chips from class lessons, she chooses to eat chips—what a radical idea. Most people have mental disorders making it difficult to stop taking some food even though we understand their repercussions on our bodies. i.e., eating chips. An article on this topic claims that most food companies are working hard at night to make fast food more addictive. According to Howard Moskovitz, a consultant in the junk food industry, they put more flavor on junk food to make you come back for more. If the food tastes too good, then we'd have what's called a sensory-specific Satia T then we wouldn't want anymore. So, companies have to find just the right balance of flavors. So, there's not too much or too little. All they do is to balance the flavors. That balance is called Bliss point.

According to Steven Weatherly, an expert in junk food, Cheetos are the core source of pleasure. They are the specific type of food manufactured by big companies to solely satisfy you and not to add any health benefit to your body. They are designed in such a manner that when you start eating them, it melts on your mouth, making it feels tasty and impressive. They are made to make you go for more. A friend was once a diet, and her boyfriend brought home Cheetos. Yes, she said no. She ended up just having one, and before she knew it, she knew almost the whole thing. Now we understand why the next log in our way we maybe think we don't like healthy food. Perhaps you don't like healthy food. You want foods that excite your palate to feel alive, be closer to something exciting, but you will not be satisfied.

You'll not reach the maximum point, and perhaps you will not know what to do. Normalizing bad habits make us feel comfortable in our negative thoughts. When you do one negative thing, the effects widely spread. Self-indulgence keeps us wrapped up in this safe place and keeps us inside of ourselves and absorbed by negative thoughts. You know, you do one thing poorly or negatively, it trickles into other areas. It leaves you feeling bad, and you do short to feel better just for the short term, such as impossible diets that you can't keep up with, and then you, you feel worse and worse about yourself and you, you go overboard when you can't keep up. It's a vicious cycle. The primary method of overcoming these key log is to fist, hit the reset button. It might not be easy, strive as much as you can by having an open mind and a positive attitude going forward.

Explore various flavors even if you don't like them. Michael's sister has a negative attitude towards blueberries. She had not consumed any since her childhood and kept telling stories that had no connection to the blueberries' taste. One day Michael made her taste the blueberry, and she loved it. Test your assumptions, test your opinions because you don't know where they came from; such an assumption may be baseless. Despite her premise on blueberries being messy, and she made a try, and she ended up loving it. Open your mind for new ideas. Remember the story of the coy and to keep figuratively throwing yourself in more significant environments, you will stretch out and grow in size. Adopt an attitude of success and stop to fetus thinking and know that your thoughts, perceptions, and behaviors can change. Why not start to look forward to fruiting and vegetables, however crazy they sound? You were not born with thoughts you possess today; they are a construct of your mind. They can be challenged.

The next solution calls for changing one's health. Saying a big NO and breaking a cycle is all you need—cutting out indulgence.

Commit yourself daily, and you'll find it easier to overcome the notion of food industries that want you to be addicted to their food. The third is growth towards what you want and the freedom you desire. This step calls for exceptional consistency. Make your bold step a pattern. This pattern will develop into the desired habit. Unpack your true self through spiritual faith and meditative silence. Strive to become better. Look inside, stop looking for solutions on the outside. Make additional efforts like being more helpful to those that are happy and caring for those that are needy, consistently reach for truth, grace, and peace in your day. Take caution on being a man of the people, and you may be living a fishy life. Finally, systems generate autonomy. We are going to be creating a system together by planning, keeping it simple, embracing balance in your life, and accomplishing these solutions and your goals by following the system to help you prioritize and reinforce consistency in your life. The best solution to weight loss is a healthy diet and an active body. There could be a reason why doing these two is a problem from your side. The pathway will make the process more holistic and more fun. All may not be your answer, but you must get something from it.

Chapter 22: Your Possible Weight Loss Block

What beliefs are holding onto your weight?

I am inferior

I am lacking

I am inconsequential, so I have to make myself big to be seen

Losing weight is too difficult

I will fail and put the weight all back on again

I must be so awful and bad not to be able to control my eating

I want to punish myself

It is too hard to start dieting

My weight is ancestral, and I can't change that

My weight is genetic, and I can't change that

I am not good enough/I am not enough

I self-sabotage myself

I am worthless

I loathe myself

Healing negative beliefs

The best ways to heal negative beliefs and build confidence are: Emotional Freedom Technique (EFTTM)–Bach Flower Remedies Affirmations

Ask your guides and angels to help heal you. A pattern is a program that you have, which is part of your personality. For example, in your personality could be the thoughts:

I am not good enough

I am useless

I can't lose weight

I am not as good as other people

I am stupid

I am ugly

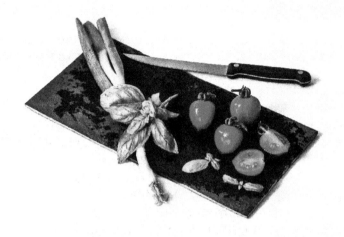

I am fat (remember if you tell yourself you are fat, you will be!)

I am to blame

It is my fault

I can't do anything right

I am a failure

This means that you block your weight loss as you feel that the task is too daunting, and you will fail. New patterns can be easily installed using EFTTM.

A block is something that stops you moving forward and the biggest one of these is FEAR. The other one is being safe. If your subconscious feels that it is not safe it WILL NOT LET YOU DO IT. So, if your subconscious feels that losing weight is not safe, you WILL NOT LOSE WEIGHT!

Also, if you think you are worthless or you feel you do not deserve, this will cause you to self-sabotage.

Healing negative patterns and blocks

The best ways to heal negative patterns and blocks are:

Emotional Freedom Technique

Bach Flower Remedies

Affirmations

Meditation

Ask your guides and angels to help heal you

What is self-sabotage?

The term, self-sabotage, describes our often-unconscious ability to stop ourselves being, doing or having; being the person we want to be, doing what we want to experience or achieve or having our goals and desires become a reality. Most of the time, we are totally unaware that we are self-sabotaging as it happens on a subconscious level. However, sometimes we are aware of that little voice in the back of our head that says, "you can't learn a language" or "don't be ridiculous, you can't lose weight."

Our subconscious mind is a powerful tool and always thinks that it is acting in our best interest. Stopping us stepping into new territory, discouraging us from taking risks ensures that we don't get hurt, we are not humiliated, and we don't fail, that is why so many projects never get off the ground. Rather than playing to win, self-sabotage plays to avoid defeat.

The purpose of this aspect of the subconscious is self-protection and survival. It can even negatively affect your health if it thinks that this will protect you from greater risk. Layers of excess weight have long been recognized as protection and very often the subconscious will use weight gain to protect you from perceived dangers you might be exposed to as a slimmer person.

For example, where someone has been abused as a child, the subconscious may add weight to make them unattractive (it thinks) so that the abuse is never repeated.

So, people may talk about self-sabotage in regard to their weight because they eat emotionally and put on weight. However, sometimes self-sabotage will affect your hormones and/or organs, causing weight gain in people who eat only a modest amount. Sometimes people can lose weight but always put it back on just another method of self-sabotage. Once the perceived need to protect through self-sabotage has been healed and released, our illnesses and weight may disappear.

My experience of self-sabotage

In my personal quest to lose the weight and water I had accumulated, I consulted a lady who specialized in 'muscle testing.' When we asked the question "Do I want to be slim," the clear reply was "no!" which took me totally by surprise. So then started the journey of discovery as to why my subconscious didn't want me to be slim.

Why was I self-sabotaging?

During the long seventeen years in which I slowly cleared and healed the reasons for my self- sabotage:

I had set up a self-punishment/self-destruct program because of what I had done in past lives

I had set up a protection around me (weight and water) because of the sexual abuse, date rape and male attention I had. I didn't feel it was safe to be a woman

I had several past life issues with starving to death and didn't want to starve in this lifetime

I had several past life issues with dying of thirst, hence the excess water in this lifetime to ensure that it didn't happen again

I had a tremendous amount of other karma

I thought that if I became a therapist I could not trust myself not to hurt, or experiment on patients, as I had hurt them before in past lives and so I was only going to be a therapist when I was 'slim'

I was frightened to take herbs as I had seen so many people die from them in past lives

Because I had been persecuted in past lives for healing people, I thought I would be persecuted in this life as well

I was frightened of being powerful

I was frightened to do the work I was supposed to do

I was frightened that the book would fail

Although I relate to my self-sabotage with weight and health there were many other areas of my life that affected.

I was always in debt and could never pay off my credit cards

I never got the job I deserved and was very often out of work

If I got a job, there would always be someone giving me a tough time (karmic payback!)

When I had any treatments, such as red vein treatment or plastic surgery, it would always go wrong

Believe it or not, my subconscious was creating a reality where all of the above occurred, the subconscious is that strong, believe me.

Even when I had released the attachments, and got rid of the influence of my mother, my subconscious was still following their examples and as I strived to get better, my subconscious really kicked in and made it worse.

So, my subconscious was actually affecting all my organs and making them work inefficiently so that I put on six stone and swelled up with water. This was because my subconscious knew I could lose weight and it decided this was the best plan of attack.

That's why some people lose weight and then put it back on. The subconscious doesn't always realize what is happening to begin with, hence the weight loss. It then kicks in big time in survival mode and the weight goes back on. You would not lose six stone and then put it back on again, you might put back a stone and then get it off. People blame diets or losing it too quickly but, in fact, it is simply your subconscious sabotaging you.

Emotional and comfort eating

When you read magazine articles they always talk about emotional eating and weight gain. Some people do eat for emotional reasons and boredom. Some people do overeat and there are explanations for this. You need to identify your emotional eating triggers and use a technique such as EFTtm to eliminate them. However, if you want to eat, try to wait for a 10-minute period breathing deeply and you should find that after that, the need to eat has gone.

However, I know a lot of slim people who overeat and drink too much. They overeat for emotional reasons as well, slim people aren't perfect or without their own problems.

Overweight people do not eat emotionally any more than slim/normal people. How often are you on holiday and you watch people eat an enormous breakfast, followed by an enormous lunch and then three courses for dinner, plus booze, every day for two weeks? How often do you see a slim person eat a packet of biscuits or a bar of chocolate? ALL THE TIME!

You have to find the reasons why your subconscious doesn't want to lose weight and either release the reasons if these are past lives based or change your subconscious 'belief system' if they are more personality traits.

Removing the self-sabotage

When I was spending a huge amount of money with therapists

and nothing worked, I did mention that I might be self-sabotaging myself. Most of them threw their hands up in horror and told me it was just an excuse to overeat (here we go again, I thought).

I read a lot about Emotional Freedom Technique (EFTTM) and in the very first paragraph, I read it mentioned self-sabotage. This was quite amazing. However, my self-sabotage was so deeply ingrained that for a long time, EFTTM just made everything worse, as my subconscious tried to hold onto its control of me.

I, therefore, had to dig much deeper by clearing the attachments, past lives, and karma and then I could use EFTTM and my other techniques to change my subconscious perception and its belief system that "I did not deserve."

Psychological reversal

I thought I wanted to lose weight, but I actually didn't and my subconscious was stopping me. You need to find out all the reasons why and release and heal them one by one. For this, you use the EFTTM psychological reversal techniques.

How are you self-sabotaging because my experience would lead me to believe that you are?

Habit of self-sabotage

I had a spiritual reading session and was told that the self-punishment had been healed but that I still had the 'habit' and that needed to be healed and not recreated. Our body and subconscious sabotage us so much that it becomes automatic and then a habit. So even when the original stimuli are healed, the habit remains. So, remember to test to see whether there is a habit and then heal accordingly (normally the same way you healed the original pattern). Make sure you don't recreate the habit by repeating affirmations and if you feel yourself slipping back into 'deserving the pattern' immediately cancel this feeling and ensure that you keep healing it.

Chapter 23: The Importance of Genetics

How You Were Raised, Counts

Those who have been overweight all their lives go through certain cycles. There is a period of unhealthy habits, the recognition that there needs to be a change, an attempt at reform, the failure to follow through, and then back to a period of unhealthy habits. This cycle is present in many people that are overweight, but for those that were overweight kids and teens, it might be better understood. We might have also adopted this unhealthy cycle from our parents. Once we've found ourselves in this dangerous position, it can feel like clawing our way out when we decide we want to lose weight. If the pattern of behavior is not at first recognized, then we won't be able to determine the best method of breaking this unhealthy habit.

Studies have proven that kids who were weight-shamed go through cycles of binge eating and meal skipping that leads to self-loathing. A child that experiences criticism from their parents will start learning unhealthy methods of coping with weight and dieting. Eating is something that we've been doing all our lives, so the way that we eat now is undoubtedly related to the way that we used to be taught to eat. Parents that might have body-shamed their kids by telling them they needed to lose weight or stop eating so much are responsible for causing self-loathing later in life.

Weight-shaming is not just blatantly telling someone that they are fat. It might also cloud diet encouragement. If your mom or dad always told you to try out a diet or suggested that you shouldn't eat a particular food, which was probably enough for you to feel a certain amount of shame about your weight. Even having a parent that continually talks about dieting is likely to make a child feel as though they should diet, too.

Many kids might grow up with moms who are always trying out new diets and fads. By seeing this is a kid, we end up going through the same phases. Maybe a parent was always saying things like, "I need to start my diet on Monday." This idea gets it in the kid's head that diets are something they should aim for, but only at a moment of convenience. The way a parent or even older sibling always talked about their body will play into how you

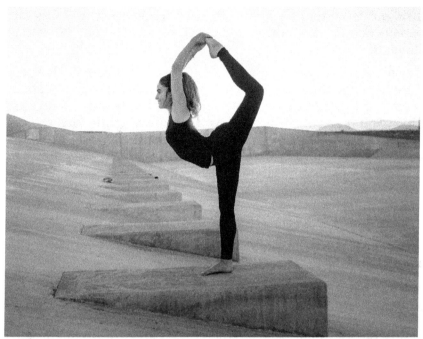

might see your own body now. Perhaps your mom was still saying things like, "I hate my thighs; they are so big!" If a girl looks in the mirror and sees she has the same shaped thighs as her mother, she'll end up thinking about how both she and her mother see those thighs as significant, even though the mother never said anything directly to the girl about her body.

It is challenging because most parents think they are helping. Parents that stock the fridge with Diet Coke instead of regular might think they are doing everyone a favor when really, they are still supplying a form of addiction. Those that make sure to weigh their kids or track their workout routines could be doing so just because they want to make sure their kid is healthy. Still, they might not realize they are setting them up in a fearful manner in which dieting and exercising are an authoritative issue. Parents who are strict with routines might raise kids that don't have any method at all as an act of rebellion.

How our parents' diet, exercise, and talk about health, in general, will also form our body perceptions. A daughter of a mother who consistently crashes diets and works out too hard will likely produce a daughter that does the same. A father that only eats microwave meals or fast food is setting his kids up for doing the same when they become adults. When this happens, it is an insidious issue that we might not even recognize. The things our parents do can seem normal to us, as it is behavior that we learn is standard.

Be mindful of how you talk about exercise around children. Whether they are your kids or someone else's, never talk about body issues around kids. If you walk around talking about how much you hate your belly flab, you are teaching the kids around you to evaluate their stomachs, wondering if they, too, have too much belly flab. Kids will be confronted with these body issues in other ways, as it is inevitable. As parents, caretakers, or any role models, we should be teaching our kids how to love their bodies and adequately take care of them because they deserve to be healthy, not because they should be skinnier or prettier.

Pregnant Moms Who Exercise Will Likely Give Birth to Healthy Kids

A study was conducted in which one group of pregnant rats were given exercise wheels, while another group of pregnant rats wasn't assigned anything. Those who used the exercise wheels ended up giving birth to more active babies. The babies of the moms that didn't work out would sit around and not do anything, as opposed to the babies of the moms that were always using an exercise wheel, who would use the wheel themselves. This was true for at least half of the rats born from active mothers. They weren't given anything else, so there weren't any factors to determine the difference in the level of activity other than the environment in which they were raised in the womb.

This exercise was inspired by similar research done on humans, though many scientists wonder if the effects were just because of a mother's influence after birth. Instead of assuming that it was from active pregnancy, many scientists speculate that the difference in the amount of desire for physical activity is because mothers with active pregnancies are also mothers with busy lives. Their lifestyle and habits can affect children, but the study with the rats proves that it might be on a level different than just the learned behavior.

Even in the womb, our mothers are teaching us how to exercise. We learn before we're also walking how vital exercise is in maintaining a high level of physical activity. If a mother is more active while she's pregnant, she's setting her unborn baby up for a future in which it is just generally more productive. This means that not only are we affected by the learned habits of our parents, but how we are actually created and grown also determines how much physical activity we let into our life.

Look back on your mother, father, or any other person that helped raise you, biologically or not. Were they active? Did they let that level of activity negatively affect your life? Did they reject exercise and healthy eating at all costs? Did you learn your unhealthy eating habits, or are they just a product of not being taught anything at all? We are taught how to eat and exercise, which means we are also taught how not to eat healthily or use. We can't entirely blame our parents for the way we live now, but it is still essential to recognize as it'll help bring us closer to closure with the unhealthy person in our head.

This is the right motivation for any woman hoping to get pregnant in the future. Starting a family is a goal for many different people. An essential aspect of starting that family is making sure to have a high level of physical activity. Kids require a lot of chasing and lifting. It is much harder for those that are not in shape to look after and give proper attention to active kids. It is also essential to be healthy when pregnant with them to get them started right away with a healthy lifestyle. After kids are born, parents are also responsible for making sure their kids understand how to live a healthy lifestyle that does not include any bad habits.

Chapter 24: How to Eat Right with The Help of Meditation

Eat fruits

When was the last time you went to the market with the intention of specifically buying fruits? You find that we purchase all other types of food, but we barely think of buying fruits. The good thing about fruits is that they are healthy, and they have plenty of nutritious benefits. If you are the type of person that loves sweet things, fruits can act as a good replacement. When consumed, they add value to your body and can prevent you from acquiring some diseases. Fruits also contain some minerals that are essential to your body. Now the question we have at the moment is how mediation will help you in taking the fruits. One of the benefits of meditating is that it allows you to differentiate between right and wrong. Eating fruits is beneficial to your body, and hence it is a good move to take.

Avoid processed foods

Currently, we are having a lot of processed foods. The food industry has been one of the fastest-growing industries. As the industry expands, the market becomes competitive, and more people join the industry. We are having new foods being introduced to the market as companies look forward to growing and gaining recognition. One of the common factors among all the companies is that they aim at pleasing the consumers. After carefully studying the target market, they know what each individual requires, which helps them in the production of their various items. If they are targeting a market with low purchasing power, they make products that are cheap and enticing. Some of the processed foods made by such companies contain a lot of chemicals and have harmful effects on the individual. You find that such foods are not helpful and only result in harm. These are the types of foods that we need to avoid if we wish to have good health. One of the things that you require for you to avoid such foods is discipline. It allows you to make the right decisions regarding what you consume, and you only take in what is helpful.

Avoid carbohydrates

In every meal that you take, you only require a small portion of carbohydrates. In most cases, we do the contrary and have the biggest percentage of our meal as a carbohydrate. When we go to this, our body receives more that it can utilize. One of the main purposes of consuming carbohydrates is that they provide us with energy. When they are consumed in excess, not all can be used to provide energy. The excess can be turned into fatty tissues, and one ends up adding some weight. In some cases, the carbohydrates can result in some diseases like cardiovascular diseases. To avoid weight gain and such diseases, it is better if one avoids taking large amounts of carbohydrates. Ensure that you only take the recommended portions. You also find that some of these foods, like bread, contain certain addictive substances. In the process, all you want to do is keep wanting to take more. As a result, you take up more than your body needs, and the excess does not benefit it in any. Mediation can help you attain some self-control. You get to eat the amount of food that your body requires.

Eating the recommended portion of food

Eating right can mean taking the amount of food that one needs. You find that certain chronic eating disorders prevent us from eating as we should. An individual with bulimia tends to consume more food than the required portion. There are various factors that can cause an individual to do so. For instance, they might be struggling with low self-esteem due to how they look. Some petite individuals wish they were a little bit bigger. As a result of their esteem issues, they end up consuming more than the required amount of food. There is a certain belief within them that if they eat a lot, they will get to the size they want. Sadly, that is not always the case. At times their body experiences no change, which can cause an individual to be frustrated. The same applies to eat less than the required amount of food. Skipping some meals is not good. You end up causing more harm to your body when you should be taking proper care of it. The best thing to do is to ensure that you take the recommended amount. This ensures that you stay healthy and fit. With the aid of mediation, you can maintain focus.

Consuming plant-based meals

Everyone should turn to eat vegetables. Plant-based meals contain nutrients that are helpful to our bodies. Some of the minerals present to ensure that our bodies are functioning as they should and normal body processes are being conducted well. The nutrients are effective in ensuring that we maintain good health by providing minerals that prevent certain diseases. Some of these minerals help in boosting the various metabolic processes occurring in our bodies. In case you have not been consuming plant-based meals, you have been missing a lot. Plant-based meals are also effective in weight loss. They ensure that we take only the right food portion that is helpful to our bodies. When most people want to start a weight loss journey, the immediate solution is talking plant-based meals. They have proven to be beneficial in that journey and process. In the past, people used to live long and were healthy because of consuming such diets. At this time, people would eat what they planted or what they hunted. They ate right and led a healthy life. One needs some discipline for them to eat plant-based meals.

Eat lightly cooked food

When we overcook meals, they do not have nutritious benefits to our bodies. You find that all the nutrients that were present are lost in the process. As you consume that food, it is not helpful to your body. Foods are beneficial when raw or when lightly cooked. Not everyone might manage to eat the foods when they are in this state. One needs some certain level of discipline for them to lightly cook their food and consume it in that state. At times you find that it is easier to consume food when fully cooked, especially with the taste that comes with it. You want to eat something sweet and something that you can easily chew. The problem with such desires is that the food will not help you in any way. At times you are torn between enjoying your meal or eating right. The two are difficult choices to choose from, and you may find yourself opting to enjoy your meal. Eating healthy can be fun, only if you tune your mind into it. Meditation will help you maintain focus, and you will easily accomplish the goals that you have set.

Reduce your sugar intake

Sugars are sweet and enticing. They make you want to eat more, and you simply cannot have enough of them. At times you crave to eat something that is sweet to your taste buds. The problem is the effect that these sugars have on your body. You find that when you consume them in excess, they cannot be utilized by the body. Instead of being converted into energy, they are converted into fats. When this happens, it can result in further complications to your body. We have some diseases such as diabetes that result from consuming excessive sugars. We also have some challenges, such as tooth problems that result from consuming sugars. At times they can be addictive, and all we wish to do is to take more of them. However, with the right discipline, we can regulate our sugar consumption. You can decide that you will be taking only a certain amount of sugars in a day. Meditation allows you to be focused on what you do. In this case, your focus is on regulating the number of sugars that you take. With this, you get to consume that which is necessary. In the end, it ensures that you have good health and that your body is in the right shape.

Avoid overeating

Overeating is a bad eating habit that everyone should avoid. In the process of overeating, one gets to add extra weight, and it has some harmful effects on their body. Mindful eating is essential in ensuring that we maintain good health. An individual's ability to focus can help them know when they are full. Different foods have different food components. There are some foods that will make you feel full at a fast rate than others will. You can analyze how your body feels after eating certain types of foods and know the effect of each food. This analysis helps you determine the portion that you should consume depending on the type of food involved. As a result, you make better and more informed decisions in terms of what you consume and watch the quantity that you take. To effectively follow this, one requires self-control that ensures they stick to the plan. This may appear like a challenging thing to accomplish, but it is possible with the help of meditation. You only need to tune your mind into consuming that which is necessary.

Chapter 25: Eating Mindlessly

We eat mindlessly. The principal explanation behind our awkwardness with nourishment and eating is that we have overlooked how to be available as we eat. Careful eating is the act of developing a receptive familiarity with how the nourishment we eat influences one's body, sentiments, brain, and all that is around us. The training improves our comprehension of what to eat, how to eat, the amount to eat, and why we eat what we eat. When eating carefully, we are completely present and relish each chomp connecting every one of our faculties to really value the nourishment. Past simple tastes, we see the appearance, sounds, scents, and surfaces of our nourishment, just as our mind's reaction to these perceptions.

The precepts of care apply to careful eating too; however, the idea of careful eating goes past the person. It likewise incorporates how what you eat influences the world. When we eat with this comprehension and understanding, appreciation and empathy will emerge inside us. Accordingly, careful eating is fundamental to guarantee nourishment supportability for who and what is to come, as we are persuaded to pick nourishments that are useful for our wellbeing, yet in addition useful for our planet.

It is outstanding that most get-healthy plans do not work in the long haul. Around 85% of individuals with heftiness who shed pounds come back to or surpass their underlying load inside a couple of years. Binge eating, passionate eating, outside seating, and eating because of nourishment longings have been connected to weight put on and weight recovers after effective weight reduction. Interminable presentation to stress may likewise assume an enormous job in gorging and heftiness. By changing the manner in which you consider nourishment, the negative sentiments that might be related to eating are supplanted with mindfulness, improved poise, and positive feelings. At the point when undesirable eating practices are tended to, your odds of long-haul weight reduction achievement are expanded.

Steps to Mindful Eating

1. Watch your shopping list

Do shopping mindfully, purchasing sound nourishments that are reasonably delivered and bundled is a significant piece of the training. One thing you will probably find about careful eating is that entire nourishments are more dynamic and heavenly than you may have given them acknowledgment for.

2. Figure out how to Eat Slower

Eating gradually does not need to mean taking it to limits. All things considered, it is a smart thought to remind yourself, and your family, that eating is not a race. Setting aside the effort to relish and make the most of your nourishment is perhaps the most advantageous thing you can do. You are bound to see when you are full, you'll bite your nourishment more and consequently digest it all the more effectively, and you'll likely end up seeing flavors you may some way or another have missed.

3. Eat when Necessary

It might take some training, however, locate that sweet spot between being eager and being ravenous to the point that you need to breathe in a dinner. Additionally, tune in to your body and get familiar with the distinction between being physically eager and sincerely ravenous. On the off chance that you skip dinners, you might be so anxious to get anything in your stomach that your first need is filling the void as opposed to making the most of your nourishment.

4. Enjoy your Senses

The vast majority partner eating with simply taste; and many eat so carelessly that even the taste buds get quick work. Be that as it may, eating is a blessing to a greater number of faculties than simply taste. When you are cooking, serving, and eating your nourishment, be mindful of shading, surface, fragrance, and even the sounds various nourishments make as you set them up. As you bite your nourishment, take a stab at distinguishing every one of the fixings, particularly seasonings. Eat with your fingers to give your feeling of touch some good times. By drawing in various faculties, the entire experience turns out to be significantly more completely fulfilling.

5. Keep off Distractions

Our day by day lives are brimming with interruptions, and it is normal for families to eat with the TV booming or one relative or another tinkering with their iPhone. Think about making family supper time, which should, obviously, be eaten together, a hardware-free zone. This does not mean eating alone peacefully; careful eating can be a great mutual encounter. It just means you do not eat before the TV, while driving, on the PC, on your telephone, and so on. Eating before the TV is for all intents and purposes the national hobby, however, simply consider how effectively it empowers careless eating.

6. Stop when you are Full

The issue with astounding nourishment is that by its very nature, it tends to be difficult to quit eating. Eating gradually will enable you to feel full before eating excessively, but on the other hand, it is imperative to be mindful of segment size and tune in to your body for when it starts disclosing to you it has had enough. Gorging may feel great at the time; however, it is awkward a short time later and is commonly not beneficial for the body. With a little practice, you can locate the without flaw spot between eating enough, however not all that much.

Careful eating does not need to be an activity in super-human focus, but instead a straightforward promise to acknowledging, regarding and, most importantly, getting a charge out of the nourishment you eat each day. It very well may be drilled with serving of mixed greens or frozen yogurt, doughnuts or tofu, and you can present it at home or at work. While the center turns out to be the means by which you eat, not what you eat, you may discover your thoughts of what you need to eat moving significantly for the better as well.

Meditating to Heal your Relationship with Food

The capacity to hold a wide scope of various feelings for the duration of the day is a test for a considerable lot of us. We simply need to feel upbeat, yet the test is to locate that mystical parity of all that we experience, decipher and do. The most regular history of past weight reduction endeavors is ceaseless confinements, which requires self-discipline and force. This perspective has a negative turn and does not draw out the best of us.

Meditation is a very accommodating device to mend enthusiastic eating. Meditation enables you to interface with your body. When you are in a condition of quiet and stillness, your state draws out the outer commotion of the world. Without these interruptions, it ends up simpler for you to drop into your body, construct, and support that association. When you have a solid association with your body, you are ready to accomplish things like unravel between physical yearning prompts versus enthusiastic appetite signals and perceive how to utilize nourishment for wellbeing and craving.

Stillness and predictable introduction to it enables you to construct your well of inward harmony and guidance. You will start to comprehend that you can exist outside of nourishment, weight, and everything in the middle. The more you reflect, the simpler you will discover it to drop into your body and associate with your higher self. You will be less inclined to go to binge eating as an approach to adapt to pressure and torment.

Meditation enables you to sharpen and use your breath. Breath resembles an inherent unwinding framework that you approach each moment of consistently. Breathing is the fastest method to accomplish a state change, which is the thing that your body is looking for when you voraciously consume food. Reflecting will condition you to depend on your breathing more on and then some, which means you will go after the shoddy nourishment less and less.

Make this a normal practice; ensure you do it consistently first and foremost. Since at that point, the requirement for nourishment to fill this hole of the void will not be as large as you discover delight from other progressively self-engaging sources. Mindfulness will develop and you will not just begin investigating yourself and your very own inward discussion, you will likewise expand your capacity to deal with the external mess. Obviously, it accepts practice likewise with each new routine, but it can likewise mend your association with nourishment.

Chapter 26: Consider Incorporating Working Out to Your Routine

The Rules of Working Out

That said, when you get going on a new exercise regimen, there are a few things you can keep in mind. These will help you get started and make sure you get the right kind of workout to suit your needs.

Firstly, the type of exercise you select will make a huge difference. To target your whole body, you need to be able to pick out a wide range of workouts. Cardio is the first form and you should spend three to four days a week getting some of this into your routine as it increases your heart rate and makes sure your heart gets some of the treatment it needs. Plus, the weight loss is really great because you can burn a lot of calories in the process.

That doesn't mean certain forms of workouts aren't important. Weight lifting can also be done a couple of days a week because it also strengthens those muscles. Your metabolism will burn much faster during the day while doing normal activities, when the muscles are toned up. So, while you may not burn as many calories as you do with cardio during the actual workout part, weight lifting can be amazing for the metabolism benefits.

And on stretching you can't forget. Take some time off your days, and do some stretching, like yoga or some other technique. This can help give the muscles a good time to relax after having worked so hard during the week, make them stronger and leaner and prevent injury.

Now, when it comes to how long you're supposed to work out, that will vary. When you want to lose weight, it's recommended you work out at least three days a week for 45 to 60 minutes. However, some people prefer to work out at whatever minutes for five or six days, so it's easier to fit into their schedule. When you are just beginning your fitness routine and it's been a while since you've worked out, beginning slowly would be better. Ten minutes is better than nothing and from there, you can build up. Never say you don't have time to work out; you can fit three or four ten-minute sessions into the day, and you've completed a full workout once you've done it.

Make sure the workouts you select have a lot of variety. Mix the stretching, cardio, and weight-lifting days together. Test out a host of different things, including some you've never done before. Mixing it up helps to focus on various muscle groups that help with weight loss and can make your workout easier to enjoy.

What if I don't have time to work out?

Some people worry they wouldn't have time to work out. They imagine spending hours at the gym to get the extra exercise you need to really see the results you like. Yet you don't need to waste all this time in the gym with Successful weight loss program. You just need to work out a few days a week, and then find other ways to fit into your routine a little bit of exercise. Some of the easy ways you can add to your routine in more movement include: Get up every hour, rather than sitting at your desk all day long and never moving, consider getting up every hour for at least two to five minutes. Walk around the room, do some jumping jacks and run around just a bit. For five minutes of an eight-hour day every hour, you'll end up for forty-five minutes of exercise. You too should bring this around. Do some sit-ups and pushups during commercial breaks during your favorite show and you will get an additional fifteen to twenty minutes each hour.

Park further away, if you need to take your vehicle, make sure you park far from the entrance. It might be just a few extra measures, but you do it a few times a day, and it really adds up.

Working out during your lunch break can be one of the best choices you can make. You can spend your lunch break just twenty minutes, and then enjoy a nutritious meal for the rest. This won't take too much of your time, so it can be a nice way to stroll around the office or work in the local gym without adjusting too much your schedule.

Take the stairs—if you're working in an office just below the first floor, try going up the stairs instead of the elevator. If the office is too far up to walk, start with a few flights and then take the rest of the way up the elevator. With time, you'll be able to increase your endurance and go up more flights of stairs.

Learn chair exercises, if you can't get up from your chair at work too often, learn a few basic exercises that will help you to work out your body without moving too often.

Add moves to chores—just cleaning the house can make you all sweaty. Make the movement intentional and add some things to it, and you're sure you'll get the additional exercise you want while making the house look fine.

Play at the park, take your kids to the park (walk there if you can) and then play at the park. Using the monkey bars, ride them, go down the slides and more. You'll be shocked to see how much of a workout this will end up for you.

There's still time to add more exercise to your day; for that to happen, you just need to be a little creative. If you get up more often from your chair or sneak a few times during the day in the workouts, you're sure to get the results you want.

The Benefits of Working Out

There are plenty of perks you'll reap when it comes to working out. You'll see a huge difference in the way your body behaves and responds, you'll be able to lower your stress levels and your attitude will begin to feel better in no time. Only ten minutes a day will make a major difference in the overall way you feel. Some of the great benefits you'll be able to see when you start working out include:

Better mood—it's time to have a workout on those days when you're just mad at everyone and grumpy... Even if you feel down and down, it's time to get out there and enjoy a good workout. Ten to fifteen minutes is all you need to make your mood feel better, and if you can work out for longer, you'll find that your body feels so much happier and satisfied when it's over.

Clearer mind—there's just something to figure out that will clean the mind out and make you feel so much better. When you feel foggy or you simply can't get any more work done for the day, and its only lunchtime, think about going out there and going into a good workout.

Healthier heart—your heart still wants some exercise. At least a few times a day, you want to use cardio to help the heart get up there and really get stronger. Also, if you have to start slowly, you will find in the beginning that working your heart with some good workouts like walking, running, swimming and cycling will help you get that heart in shape.

Faster weight loss—you eat calories while you work out. So, the more calories you eat up, the faster the weight loss becomes. Your metabolism should be quicker, and it can eat up all the excess fat the remains in the body, so you'll be able to see some of those weight loss results quicker than ever before.

Toned muscles—sitting on the couch doesn't help your muscles be safe and strong. Instead, it makes them frail and fragile and waste away. Neither do you just have to focus on weight lifting; stretching and cardio also have those muscles up and going, and you can see more strength in your body. Besides, these toned muscles will help speed up the metabolism, which is good whether or not you choose to lose weight.

Leaves you want more—beginning on an exercise plan may seem difficult at the beginning, and you may want to go out and do something else, you will learn to love it. If you can only keep up with the job for some time, you can see some amazing results in the process. You'll start looking forward to the workout, for instance, to see how many results you can achieve. If you're someone who gets bored with the workout, just have a plan every few months or so to change it and you're going to be perfect.

Although many people hate working out and putting all the time into it, there is actually a lot of good that can come from daily exercise. Give it a chance together with the other parts of your Successful weight loss program plan to see how much the outcomes will improve.

Chapter 27: Banning Food

The entire approach of intuitive eating revolves around listening to the body and keeping a finger on its pulse. If you are unable to follow the signals your body is giving out properly, then you are going to face problems in implementing this lifestyle. Any dietician that you go to initially or talk about with on the subject of intuitive eating will tell you that it's based on recognizing hunger and satisfying the needs accordingly. Earlier on, you read how there are different kinds of desire, and what you feel at times is not always what it seems like. Most of us are only familiar with physical hunger and spend our lives believing that it's the only type that exists.

The healthy living approach of intuitive eating has informed every one of us that this is not the case. Your body experiences varying forms of hunger, and they do not always have to be satisfied with the consumption of food. One of the first core principles of this philosophy teaches people to honor their hunger. This is about being aware of the biological urge which asks you to eat and then stop when you no longer feel empty. People say that at times, this can get confusing as, during the initial stages, one is still trying to train their body and mind. If you think about it, exploring where and what kind of hunger may not be as difficult as one would assume.

There are no technicalities or complications which you have to unravel. Just consider these few points:

• When you feel hungry, wherein your body can handle the physical sensation? Are your stomach wrenching and gnawing? If not, does your throat itch for something? Do you feel sluggish and tired? Sometimes, you might not experience any such thing but instead, start feeling weak and experiencing a headache. If this happens out of nowhere, it's a sign that your body needs to be replenished with nutrients.

• Does hunger affect your mood or concentration? Do you find yourself thinking of food in the middle of work or a conversation? Those who have answered yes to both these questions, well, there you have it. When you feel hungry, your mood changes for the worse, your ability to concentrate on any task hinders, and if your thoughts are going out to meals and snacks, then that is quite obvious.

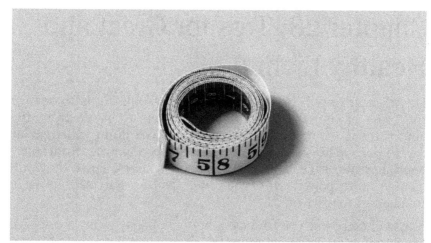

• Are there any changes in your hunger when you travel, stressed, or functioning on low sleep? To determine those, you need to closely monitor your body and try to remedy the source of the change because a disturbance in the eating pattern may be emotional hunger rather than physical.

An integral aspect here which people should be mindful of is that everyone experiences or feels hunger differently, and what one person goes through does not apply to the other. Just remember that intuitive eating has no wrong answers, and it's a practice that brings about gradual progress, so if you do not get it instantly, there is nothing wrong with that because no one ever does.

Moving on to the other hunger, which we talked about that is emotional and does not require any satisfaction, which comes from food. There are four types of desire that people generally experience; real, which you should immediately respond to according to the intuitive eating philosophy, and then emotional, practical, and taste. In the beginning, you found out what physical and emotional hunger was about and how to successfully deal with each of them. Physical hunger is perhaps the most important one here as it's your body reaching out to you and sending cues. This is also something that a lot of people fail to pay adequate attention to. You see, the diet mentality and culture has led to many treating their necessary hunger as an enemy. They consider it as a challenge which has to be overcome because otherwise, it would result in shame and guilt. Well, how can something so essential and necessary for your survival be wrong for you? Hence, when your body begins to communicate with you, learn to listen.

Chapter 28: Tips for Great and Healthy Living

The ideal approach to accomplish better wellbeing is to change your way of life. It's tied in with causing a change from the nourishments you to eat to the exercises you do in your regular day to day existence. You can begin by staying away from lousy nourishments, slick, and handled food sources, since they will include more pounds into your body just as start setting aside some effort to work out.

This will empower you to have a better capacity to burn calories, which will help consume more fats just as get your body fit as a fiddle. This is only something you can do in remaining sound. To get more direction, simply read on as right now, we share with you tips on how you can begin your way towards a more useful life and you! Appreciate!

1. Sleep for at any rate of 8 hours every night.

Having enough rest part of the most significant activities to improve and keep up your wellbeing. It can make you increasingly vigorous the following day, besides the way that it can likewise forestall binge eating. All the more significantly, it is additionally perhaps the ideal approaches to prevent diseases, since it toughens your insusceptible framework.

2. Wash your hands as often as possible.

Washing your hands for the same number of times as you can for the entire day is perhaps the most ideal approach to forestall diseases. It ought to be finished with running water and a decent antibacterial cleanser. What's more, washing ought to be accomplished for in any event 20 seconds, to guarantee that it is liberated from any malady disease germs.

3. Never skip breakfast.

If your objectives are to get more benefits and to abstain from putting on an excessive amount of weight, at that point, skipping breakfast ought to be the keep going thing on your mind. Breakfast is the essential meal of the day. The feed can prop you up all consistently. If you skip it, odds are, you will put on weight because of binge eating and limited capacity to burn calories.

4. Drink, at any rate, eight glasses of water every day.

Water can help your body in flushing out poisons. Besides that, it can likewise guarantee that you are appropriately hydrated. Besides, drinking water can also help in stifling your hunger, which results in a fitter you. In this manner, make sure that you drink at any rate eight glasses of water each day to keep up your wellbeing.

5. Limit espresso consumption.

Espresso can now and again influence the nature of your absorption, which is the reason it ought not to be drilled all the time. A great many people drink various cups of espresso every day. To get more benefits, it is ideal if you chop it down to only one container for each day, or just to make drinking espresso a trivial thing.

6. Purchase a littler plate to either chop down your weight or to look after it.

Decreasing the measure of nourishments that you eat in every meal can have an emotional impact, with regards to keeping up or shedding pounds. Something you can accomplish for it is to buy a little plate, which is for your utilization as it were. With a bit of dish, you can fool yourself into eating littler segments, which would give you bunches of medical advantages over the long haul.

7. Try not to eat whatever isn't on your plate.

To acquire control on the measure of nourishments that you eat every day, it is ideal to abstain from eating nourishment that isn't on your plate. There are loads of occasions when you might need to get a bunch of peanuts out of the holder or take a sample of soup out of the bowl with a spoon. If you keep on doing this, at that point, you include more calories into your body without knowing it.

8. Eat-in a more slow way.

Eating quick is probably the ideal way if you need to put on more weight. Like this, you are doing something contrary to that can result in losing an abundance of pounds of weight. In this way, the time has come to make the most of your meals more by eating more slowly. At the point when you eat more slowly, you can stifle your craving, and it can likewise cause you to feel full, regardless of whether you have not expended a lot of nourishments yet after a specific timeframe.

9. Be sound emotionally.

As opposed to what a few people may accept, your feelings likewise assume an incredible job with regards to your wellbeing. In this manner, it is ideal if you can oversee it. As such, attempt to forestall blowing up, and consistently attempt to have an uplifting viewpoint of life. At the point when you do this, you can get more settled in most testing circumstances.

10. Think positive.

A few people may not trust it, yet your mind can influence your wellbeing in specific manners. For instance, if you generally imagine that you are becoming ill, at that point, it will build your odds of getting influenced by an ailment. Then again, if you believe that you are stable, at that point, you become increasingly dynamic, and it would likewise support your insusceptible framework.

11. Dodge popular fashion diets.

Most craze diets are diet programs, which are intended to cause individuals to get more fit quickly. By and large, these projects can include causing the individual to experience starvation, which can result in a quicker rate in getting more fit. In any case, because of the way that it has been accomplished, you can restore the weight in merely an issue of weeks, and you may even get heavier than when you previously began with it.

12. A brisk stroll for 3 to multiple times every week.

Energetic strolling is a movement that you can appreciate with your loved ones. It can help in boosting your digestion, which can result in weight loss. Besides that, it can likewise take care of business, your hips, bottom, just as your legs. Intend to energetic stroll for at any rate 20 minutes in 3 to 4 times each week, to pick up the advantages from it.

13. Exploit practice recordings.

If you are the sort of individual who wouldn't like to invest energy in driving, to find a right pace rec center, at that point, remind yourself that there are practice recordings that you can exploit. These recordings can be played at the solaces of your home whenever you need them. You should simply follow the schedules appeared in it and appreciate them.

14. Play with your children all the more frequently

Children are so lively, and we regularly wonder why. Be that as it may, if you play with them, you can help your vitality level too. This can result in a higher metabolic rate. In this manner, it can assist you with consuming more fats and calories, besides the way that doing it all the more frequently can likewise give you an approach to bond with them more.

15. Drink a glass of water when you wake up.

Drinking a glass of water after awakening offers a ton of medical advantages. For one, it gets your framework working, which can support up your vitality level. What's more, it can likewise help in purging your assemblage of poisons that have been aggregated for a long while.

16. Sharing is something that you ought not to do in ensuring your wellbeing.

With regards to your wellbeing, sharing ought not to be finished. This relates to the sharing of your things to different people, for example, hankies, toothbrushes, nail cutters, and such. The facts demonstrate that sharing is acceptable. However, this ought not to be watched about your own things.

17. Mind your pets.

A few people don't know that there are sure ailments, which can be transmitted from creatures to people. Along these lines, if you have pets, at that point, ensure that they are given their suggested inoculations. What's more, you ought to likewise make sure that they are appropriately prepped, with the goal that they are liberated from ticks and bugs that may also convey germs.

18. Try not to confound ache to hunger.

There are times when we open up our coolers to get a bite, in any event, when our body is aching for water. This is because we tend to decipher thirst as appetite. Consequently, if you want to eat in any event, when you have quite recently had your meal, at that point, attempt to drink a glass of water. By and large, you will feel fulfilled as a result of it, particularly since you were dehydrated in any case.

19. Maintain a strategic distance from prepared nourishments as much as you can.

Handled nourishments like franks, burgers, French fries, and such don't contain enough supplements to furnish your body with what it needs. Besides that, they are likewise topped off with a ton of artificial flavorings, which can make your body amass bunches of poisons. Therefore, it is ideal for evading them for as much as you can. Staying away from them can help forestall maladies, besides the way that it would likewise help in making you more beneficial.

20. Eat nourishments that are high in fiber content.

If one of your wellbeing objectives is to shed a couple of pounds, at that point load up on fiber, fiber draws out the absorption procedure, which implies that it can cause you to feel full more. At the point when that occurs, you usually are stifling your hunger. Besides that, fiber can likewise help in freeing your assortment of waste.

21. Cut down your utilization of carbonated sodas.

Carbonated sodas are stacked with a great deal of sugar, which can make you put on weight, and it can even build your odds of getting diabetic. A few people who are partial to drinking such refreshments incline toward diet ones since they guarantee to contain lesser measures of sugar. Be that as it may, such beverages are stacked with aspartame, which can cause heaps of medical problems over the long haul.

22. Utilize the stairs rather than the lift.

At whatever point you report to your office, make it a propensity to utilize the stairs rather than the lift. This can offer an original route for you to consume more fats and calories. It is a type of activity, which can fortify your leg muscles, and it is a decent option in contrast to running or lively strolling.

23. Eat more organic products.

Organic products are stacked with natural nutrients and dampness to keep you feeling better. It is perhaps the ideal approach to forestall ailments and blockage. Most organic products additionally contain chemicals that help your body in engrossing the supplements offered by the nourishments that you eat.

Chapter 29: The Rapid Weight Loss: Good or Bad?

No nourishment is taboo when you pursue this arrangement, which doesn't make you purchase any prepackaged suppers.

Rapid Weight Loss appoints different nourishments Point esteem. Nutritious nourishments that top you off have less focuses than garbage with void calories. The eating plan factors sugar, fat, and protein into its focuses counts to direct you toward natural products, veggies, and lean protein and away from stuff that is high in sugar and immersed fat.

You'll have a Point focus on that is set up dependent on your body and objectives. For whatever length of time that you remain inside your everyday target, you can spend those Points anyway you'd like, even on liquor or treat, or spare them to utilize one more day.

However, more beneficial, lower-calorie nourishments cost less focuses. Furthermore, a few things presently have 0 points.

Level of Effort: Medium

Rapid Weight Loss is intended to make it simpler to change your propensities long haul, and it's adaptable enough that you ought to have the option to adjust it to your life. You'll improve your eating and lifestyle designs a considerable lot of which you may have had for quite a long time and you'll make new ones.

How much exertion it takes relies upon the amount you'll need to change your propensities.

Cooking and shopping: Expect to figure out how to shop, cook solid nourishments, and eat out in manners that help your weight-loss objective without holding back on taste or expecting to purchase strange nourishments.

Bundled nourishments or dinners: Not required.

In-person gatherings: Optional.

Exercise: You'll get a customized action objective and access to the program's application that tracks Points. You get acknowledgment for the entirety of your action.

Does It Allow for Dietary Restrictions or Preferences?

Because you pick how you spend your Points, you can at present

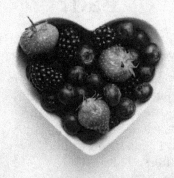

do Rapid Weight Loss if you're a veggie-lover, vegetarian, have different inclinations, or if you have to confine salt or fat.

What Else You Should Know

Cost: Rapid Weight Loss offers three plans: Online just, online with gatherings, or online with one-on-one training through telephone calls and messages. Check the Rapid Weight Loss site for the evaluation of "online just" and "online with gatherings" alternatives (you'll have to enter your ZIP code).

Costs and offers may differ.

Backing: Besides the discretionary in-person gatherings (presently called health workshops) and individual instructing, Rapid Weight Loss Program has an application, an online network, a magazine, and a site with plans, tips, examples of overcoming adversity, and that's only the tip of the iceberg.

Does It Work?

Rapid Weight Loss is one of the well-looked into weight loss programs accessible. What's more, indeed, it works.

Numerous studies have demonstrated that the arrangement can assist you with getting more fit and keep it off.

For example, an investigation from The American Journal of Medicine demonstrated that individuals making Rapid Weight Loss lost more weight than those attempting to drop beats without anyone else.

Rapid Weight Loss positioned first both for "Best Weight Loss Diet" and for "Best Commercial Diet Plan" in the 2018 rankings from U.S. News and World Report.

Generally speaking, it's a great, simple to-pursue program.

Is It Good for Certain Conditions?

Rapid Weight Loss is useful for anybody. In any case, its attention on nutritious, low-calorie nourishments makes it extraordinary for individuals with hypertension, elevated cholesterol, diabetes, and even coronary illness.

If you pick any premade dinners, check the names, as some might be high in sodium.

Please work with your primary care physician so they can check your advancement, as well. This is particularly significant for individuals with diabetes, as you may need to alter your medication as you get in shape.

If the idea of gauging your nourishment or checking calories makes your head turn, this is a perfect program because it takes every necessary step for you. The online instrument allocates a specific number an incentive to every nourishment, even eatery nourishments, to make it simple to remain on track.

If you don't have the foggiest idea about your way around the kitchen, the premade dinners and bites make it simple. They're a speedy and simple approach to control partition sizes and calories.

You don't need to drop any nourishment from your eating routine, yet you should constrain divide sizes to curtail calories.

The accentuation on foods grown from the ground implies the eating routine is high in fiber, which helps keep you full. Also, the program is easy to pursue, making it simpler to adhere to. You can likewise discover Rapid Weight Loss Program premade dinners at your neighborhood market.

A major favorable position of Rapid Weight Loss is their site. They offer exhaustive data on abstaining from excessive food intake, exercise, cooking, and wellness tips, just as online care groups.

Beset up to go through some cash to get the full advantages of the vigorous program. It tends to be somewhat expensive, yet it's well justified, despite all the trouble to harvest the wellbeing advantages of getting more fit and keeping it off.

Part Benefits

Dieters who join Rapid weight loss are known as "individuals."

Individuals can browse a few projects with differing levels of help.

An essential online program incorporates every minute of every day online visit support, just as applications and different instruments. Individuals can pay more for face to face bunch gatherings or one-on-one help from a Rapid weight loss individual mentor.

Individuals additionally get access to an online database of thousands of nourishments and plans, notwithstanding the following application for logging Points.

Also, Rapid weight loss supports physical action by relegating a wellness objective utilizing Points.

Every action can be signed into the Rapid weight loss application until the client arrives at their week after week FitPoint objective.

Exercises like moving, strolling and cleaning would all be able to be tallied towards your Point objective.

Rapid weight loss additionally gives wellness recordings and exercise schedules for their individuals.

Alongside diet and exercise directing, Rapid weight loss sells bundled nourishment like solidified suppers, cereal, chocolates and low-calorie dessert.

Outline

Rapid weight loss doles out guide esteems toward nourishments. Individuals must remain under their assigned day by day nourishment and drink focuses to meet their weight-misfortune objectives.

Would it be able to Help You Lose Weight?

Rapid weight loss utilizes a science-based way to deal with weight misfortune, accentuating the significance of part control, nourishment decisions and moderate, predictable weight misfortune.

Dissimilar to numerous craze diets that guarantee unreasonable outcomes over brief timeframes, Rapid weight loss discloses to individuals that they ought to hope to lose .5 to 2 pounds (.23 to .9 kg) every week.

The program features lifestyle modification and advice individuals on the best way to settle on better choices by utilizing the Points framework, which organizes sound nourishments.

Numerous studies have demonstrated that Rapid weight loss can help with weight misfortune.

Rapid weight loss gives a whole page of their site to scientific examinations supporting their program.

One study found that overweight individuals who were advised to get more fit by their PCPs lost twice as a lot of weight on the Rapid weight loss program than the individuals who got standard weight misfortune directing from essential care proficient.

Even though this investigation was subsidized by Rapid weight loss, information gathering, and examination were facilitated by a free research group.

Besides, an audit of 39 controlled examinations found that members following the Rapid weight loss program lost 2.6% more weight than members who got different sorts of guidance.

Another controlled investigation in more than 1,200 hefty grown-ups found that members who pursued the Rapid weight loss program for one year lost significantly more weight than the individuals who got self-improvement materials or brief weight-misfortune counsel.

Besides, members following Rapid weight loss for one year were increasingly fruitful at keeping up their weight misfortune for more than two years, contrasted with different gatherings.

Rapid weight loss is one of only a handful scarcely any weight-misfortune programs with demonstrated outcomes from randomized controlled preliminaries, which are considered the "best quality level" of therapeutic research.

Conclusion

You look in the mirror and you are dissatisfied. Do you wish that your shape, your nose, your legs, your hair were like somebody else's? Why do we always compare ourselves? Why aren't we reconciled with our appearance? We have heard ad nauseam that we should love ourselves, despite our mistakes or flaws. This includes things related to our personality as well as our bodies. However, there are very few people who can accept and be content with themselves. It is not about not wanting to change. It is a commendable endeavor when one wants to achieve or retain their looks or care about looking more attractive.

At the same time, most people are much more critical, stricter with themselves than justified. They are continuously dissatisfied with themselves and don't see in the mirror what others see. Some girls feel a significant discomfort looking at each other, both because they don't like looking at each other in general, and because they don't like what they see. Where do these reactions come from?

What usually happens is that you don't look at yourself; you only see yourself with respect to that ideal of beauty that you have in your head. This is where dissatisfaction creeps in. It has to do with the theory of social confrontation. We compare ourselves with those we consider better than ourselves; self-esteem is negatively affected. We all have a model in the head, a term of comparison that we have built by looking at years of magazines, advertising, and movies with perfect Hollywood princesses. The mantra must become one and only one: there is no need for me to compare myself to that model because everybody is a unique, generous specimen, rich in the indications of what I am.

Life would be much simpler and happier if we could accept ourselves as we are. A lot of negative emotions would be released, we would have less stress, and more of the things that really matter come into view. The bottom line is, if we really need to change something, we can't do it until we make peace with the current state. This is a vicious circle.

The mind works, in effect, in a strange way. If we resist something, we get more of it.

After all, if we focus our attention on what is bad, we reinforce the bad. And what we pay the most attention to as we think about something will come true.

Everything that comes from you that relates to you is just yours: your feelings, your voice, your actions, your ears, your thighs, your hopes and fears. That's why you are unique. Be happy that you are different from anyone, that you look the way you do and that it is just you. Start to feel that it's your own body, not something separate that you need to live with.

Do you want your house to be just like anyone else's? Or do you love the little things that carry memories? Don't you love the atmosphere of your messy place after playing with your kids? And the plain curtain that you know you should replace, but which your mom sewed and looks so good? Or the piece of furniture that everyone says you should throw out, but you insist on it?

That's how you should feel about your body. You should understand that you don't need to compare it with anyone else's because it's impossible to compare unique things. In addition, who determines what beautiful and ugly mean? You should not compare your body to the celebrities' perfect-looking bodies. First, because they are adjusted with Photoshop and other programs, and they are not real. Second, because you are different, as is everybody.

You're not them. You are neither the next-door girl who, after three children, looks like she did at twenty, nor your friend who you think is gorgeous. You should not only accept your body, but you should fall in love with it. Do you think like Bonnie? Do you think no one could love you because you have some extra weight? Then ask yourself the following questions. Could you fall in love with someone only if they are perfect looking? Would you really love someone because of their body? I'll go further.

Do we really love perfect looking people? I bet you prefer your imperfect companion instead of a perfect looking bodybuilder. You like the little faults of your wife, husband, kids, and friends because they belong to you too. We love imperfections better than perfections.

See? We don't measure people based on their weight. In addition, if you are happy with your body and your existence, it will also manifest in your radiance.

How should you love your body?

Compliment yourself. You should consider yourself and treat

yourself with the same kindness and the same admiration that you would reserve for those you love. You probably wouldn't direct the same criticisms you do to yourself, to another person. Don't hesitate to compliment yourself, don't be too hard on yourself and forgive yourself when you make a mistake. Get rid of the hatred you feel for yourself, replace it with greater understanding and appreciation. Look in the mirror and repeat: "I am attractive. I am sure of myself. I am fantastic!" Do it regularly and you'll begin to see yourself in a positive light. When you reach a goal, be proud. Look in the mirror and say, "Great job, I'm proud of myself."

Stay away from negativity. Avoid people who only talk badly about their bodies. You risk getting infected by their insecurities and dwelling on your faults. Life is too short and valuable to be consumed by hating yourself or looking for every little fault, especially when the perception you have of yourself tends to be much more critical than that of others. If a person starts to criticize their body, don't get involved in their negativity. Change the subject instead or leave. Wear comfortable clothes that reflect who you are. Everything you have in the wardrobe should enhance your body. Don't wear uncomfortable clothes just to impress others. Remember that those who accept themselves always look great. Wear clean, undamaged garments to dress the body the way you deserve. Buy matching briefs and bras, even though you are the only one to see them. You will remind your inner self that you are doing it exclusively for yourself.

Ask others what they love about you and what they consider your best qualities. This will help you develop yourself and remind you that your body has given you so much. You will probably be surprised to discover what others find beautiful about you; you have probably forgotten about them.

People, who are not inclined towards exercise and often become lazy when it comes to physical activities, will find that meditation philosophy makes it exponentially more comfortable to get started with them. It doesn't even matter whether you have exercised before in your life or not, and you can begin right from where you are! The methodology of meditating for rapid weight loss is about putting your intuition into work and trusting your 'gut.' This is not just restricted to food but applies to physical exercise and movement as well.

CPSIA information can be obtained
at www.ICGtesting.com
Printed in the USA
BVHW092316270421
605945BV00010B/1009

9 781801 779388